sleep
ARE YOU GETTING ENOUGH?

The science of sleep, and how to get more

GEORGE A.F. SEBER

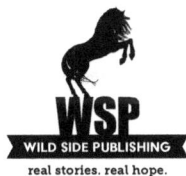

WSP
WILD SIDE PUBLISHING
real stories. real hope.

wildsidepublishing.com

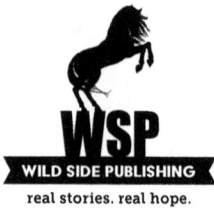

WSP

WILD SIDE PUBLISHING

real stories. real hope.

Published by George A.F. Seber in association with
Wild Side Publishing, PO Box 33, Ruawai 0549, New Zealand
wildsidepublishing.com

Cover design, Janet Curle | wildsidepublishing.com
Text layout, George A. F. Seber

Cataloguing in Publication Data:
Title: Sleep: Are you getting enough?
ISBN: 978-0-473-52504-0 (pbk)
ISBN: 978-0-473-52505-7 (epub)

Subjects: New Zealand Non-Fiction, Sleep, Health

First printing June 2020
International listing June 2020 ingramspark.com

CONTENTS (continued)

You have no doubt had occasions where you have slept badly and found yourself feeling tired, unable to concentrate, and perhaps cranky the next day. We all know when we have had inadequate sleep. In fact everyone will have spells in their lives when they have sleep problems. For example, pain will keep you awake. As a person who has had a lot of surgery I have certainly found this to be so. In fact some time ago I had a fall and broke some ribs, ending up sleeping in a chair for several weeks and having indifferent sleep.

Stress can also be a sleep stopper as the nervous system can become over sensitive. This can lead to anxiety or even a full-blown panic attack, which can happen when a person is just about to fall asleep. Their whole body goes into action with a thumping heart and very uncomfortable feelings thereby preventing sleep, because the body is ready for action.

Sometimes a person can lay awake with a problem they have been trying to solve all day, as they have taken the problem to bed with them. I know all about this as a retired professor of statistics having carried out mathematical research for decades. We all have personal problems from time to time that need sorting out or solving. Parents with babies and small children will know about interrupted nights as with shift workers or those flying to other countries and coping with changes in time zones. Looking after someone who is ill can be a sleep breaker. When my first wife was dying of cancer I had to give her morphine every four hours, which completely messed up my sleeping.

With the pace of modern living where the internet has made our lives busier instead of slower, insomnia is quite common. It is sometimes a side issue with people I meet in my counselling room. There are also a number of conditions such as sleep apnea and even someone's snoring that can disturb sleep. We may ask questions like how much sleep should I have and how long should I take a sleep medication for if I need to have it.

In this booklet I endeavour to cover all aspects of sleep including what we know scientifically about sleep and answer some questions like those just mentioned above. I will look at things to avoid when preparing for or trying to sleep and things that can be done to promote a healthful sleep. The booklet is written for anyone having sleep problems or has a friend or family member struggling with sleep issues.

Chapter 1 deals with insomnia, its physical and mental effects, why we need sleep and how much, our biological clock, and other factors such as shift working and age. Sleep cycles and various stages of sleep are considered in chapter 2, where we look at the effects of body temperature and light, and the nature of dreams. Sleep strategies are given in chapter 3 with a discussion on various topics relating to bed preparation, waking during the night, breathing techniques, sleep positions, the role of sleeping pills and natural alternatives, depression, jet lag, and cognitive behaviour therapy for sleep problems. This is backed up in the appendix with a practical programme for sleep management, as well as a brief summary of sleep disorders.

Finally, my special thanks goes to Amy Hendrickson who has allowed me to use her LATEX computer package, and has provided help on occasions.

GEORGE A. F. SEBER

Auckland, New Zealand
April, 2020

WHY SLEEP IS IMPORTANT

1.1 THE NATURE OF INSOMNIA

Sleep is universal amongst all animal creatures, even for insects and primitive worms, and is fundamental for life. Animals deprived of sleep will die. When it comes to humans we are beginning to find that adequate sleep is more important than realised in the past. Which would you regard as most important — diet, exercise, or sleep, as all three are important? Unfortunately we all have sleep problems from time to time due to a variety of circumstances. The term loosely used is *insomnia*, which refers to a difficulty in falling asleep and/or staying asleep (e.g., early morning awakening and staying awake *despite adequate opportunity and time to sleep*. The last phrase needs to be added when technically defining insomnia (see Appendix A3 for a clinical description). Other criteria include clinically significant distress or impairments in important areas of functioning (social, occupational, educational, academic, and behavioural), sleep difficulties occurring at least 3 nights per week, and present for at least 3 months. The two latter criteria are needed to distinguish insomnia from just sleep deprivation, which can occur at any time due to circumstances such as having a short time in bed or an emotional disturbance. Another criterion is that the insomnia is not attributable to the physiological effects of drug abuse or medication, and coexisting mental disorders and medical conditions do not adequately explain the predominant complaint of insomnia.

We find that insomnia can have a huge affect on a person's life. Physiologist Dr Guy Meadows, founder of London's Sleep School, said (NZ Herald, October, 2013):

> I see clients who have completely stopped living their lives in the hope of controlling their sleep. They have given up working to avoid stress, stopped socialising to avoid being out late, stopped going away on holiday or staying with family for fear of not being able to sleep in a foreign environment, and even chosen not to have children for fear of being bad parents.

Insomnia can lead to not feeling properly rested after a night's sleep, experiencing daytime fatigue, sleepiness, tension headaches, poor attention and concentration, mood changes, increased errors or accidents, and ongoing worries about sleep. Drowsy driving leads to a large number of traffic accidents and deaths every year. Insomnia is very common and is described as an epidemic throughout the industrialised nations by the World Health Organization (WHO). It affects people of all ages, including children, but is more common in adults and the elderly. Also it affects women more than men, particularly as women can have hormonal shifts during menstruation and menopause, and be sleep affected during pregnancy. Sleep data show that women average about 20 minutes more sleep per night than men until the age of about 45, at which point the gap narrows. Insomnia is more prevalent in middle-aged or older adults, shift workers, and patients with medical and psychiatric diseases. In young adults, difficulties of sleep initiation are more common; in middle-aged and older adults, problems of maintaining sleep are more common.

1.1.1 Temporary or persistent

Insomnia can be temporary (acute) due to a variety of circumstances such as jet lag, shift work, stressful life situations lasting up to a month (e.g., divorce, death of someone close, losing a job, having a new job, and having concerns about work, school, and health or family). This type of insomnia typically resolves when the stressor is no longer present or the individual adapts to the stressor. Then there is persistent (chronic) insomnia which can be due to poor sleep habits or an underlying physical or psychological problem. Acute insomnia can last for a few days or weeks while chronic insomnia can last for a month or more. In the past most cases of chronic insomnia were regarded as secondary to another primary medical or psychiatric condition. However, it should be noted that Chawla (2018) in an extensive and helpful article said:

> insomnia often persists despite treatment of the primary condition, and in certain cases, persistence of insomnia can increase the risk of relapse of the primary condition. Thus, clinicians need to understand that insomnia is a condition in its own right that requires prompt recognition and treatment to prevent morbidity and improve patients' quality of life.

Here the primary condition is some health issue other than insomnia.

1.2 SLEEP AND HEALTH

Persistent loss of sleep can have a major affect on our brain and physical wellbeing. For example, Dr Matthew Walker, a professor of neuroscience and psychology at University of California, linked persistent sleep loss to a long list of conditions such as (Walker, 2018, p.133 and his chapter 8) anxiety, depression, bipolar disorder, suicide, stroke, chronic pain, post-traumatic stress disorder, cancer, overeating, blood sugar increase and type 2 diabetes, breathing or heart problems, calcification of the coronary arteries, high blood pressure, immune system compromised, overactive sympathetic nervous system causing stress, overeating and obesity (even with young children), acid reflux, thyroid problems, urinary problems, reproductive decline in males and females, Parkinson's disease, post-traumatic stress disorder, and dementia (including Alzheimer's disease). Phew! I hope I haven't scared the reader with such a long list, but I do want to emphasise the wide variety of problems that can arise from under-sleeping. In general, a major psychiatric condition can cause sleep problems while poor sleep may lead to some psychiatric conditions—a two-way process. One of the most notorious brain toxins linked to Alzheimer's disease (AD) is amyloid-beta. This protein is responsible for forming the plaque associated with AD. It is removed from the brain far more effectively than usual while we have deep Non Rapid Eye Movement sleep (NREM sleep; section 2.1). Therefore it would appear that inadequate sleep is a key lifestyle factor determining whether or not one gets AD. Clearly the two are linked. More generally, a major psychiatric condition can cause sleep problems while poor sleep may lead to some psychiatric conditions—a two-way process. After a bad night you might feel you have got all of the above health problems! What is perhaps surprising is that it does not take much of a sleep change, e.g., one hour with daylight saving, to affect things like the number of traffic accidents and rates of heart attacks in society.

Some of the health problems previously mentioned may be debatable as causality is not readily determined, but the connection is there. It is not easy to build in lifestyle factors with epidemiological data, which is the case with the debate on alcohol and its so-called cardio-vascular support. For example, a study by Kripke, Langer, and Kline (2012), in studying sleep hypnotics with respect to cancer or mortality, adjusted the data for age, gender, smoking, body mass index, ethnicity, marital status, alcohol use and prior cancer. Even then the authors reported that:

> The major limitation was that residual confounding could not be fully
> excluded, due to possible biases affecting which patients were prescribed
> hypnotics and due to possible imbalances in surveillance.

In other words, it is clearly not easy to allow for a range of personal factors. In addition to epidemiological studies, sleep experiments are of course helpful, but sophisticated equipment may be needed, thus limiting the sample size. Also many experiments are carried out under laboratory conditions, with people becoming like "lab rats", instead of being studied under "normal" conditions during a normal day of activities. However, such experiments are valuable and have led to many insights about sleep.

1.3 NEW ZEALAND SCENE

New Zealand's National Health Survey 2013-2014 revealed that 37 per cent of Kiwis aged 30-60 never, or rarely, get enough sleep. An extensive study carried out by Wilsmore et al. (2013) using 22,389 people aged 16-84 who volunteered to donate blood found that 60% would like more sleep, and 45% reported suffering the symptoms of insomnia at least once a week. The study concluded that

> Even in a large, relatively young and healthy sample, sleep dissatisfaction,
> inadequate sleep duration, insomnia, and excessive daytime sleepiness are
> common.

Clearly the number of people recorded as having insomnia will depend on how the degree of insomnia is defined and how often it occurs, but it is clearly a major problem. Also, in New Zealand, we seem to have some ethnic differences with, for example, Maori being affected more than non-Maori (Paine, Gander, et al., 2005).

A New Zealand sleep expert, Professor Phillippa Gander, is reported as saying

> We really have a huge problem with insomnia in New Zealand. A big part of this is a failure to recognise, at all levels of society, politically, medically, the importance of sleep.

As director of the Massey university's sleep/wake research centre, she said that the funding available in the New Zealand healthcare system for the treatment of insomnia is zero, and services for people with sleep disorders were woefully inadequate. Some people boast about how little they sleep and even equate extra sleep with laziness! In the workplace insufficient sleep is commonly tolerated and even encouraged even if other health policies (e.g., smoking) are put in place. However Professor Gander said:

> We need to drop this idea that to get more out of a busy life we can cut back on sleep. You can't just expect that a third of your life doesn't matter and expect that everything else will go fine. Sleep is an essential part of being fully human.

Walker (2018:303) makes the telling comment:

> Allowing and encouraging employees, supervisors, and executives to arrive at work well rested turns them from simply looking busy yet ineffective, to being productive, honest, useful individuals who inspire, support, and help each other.

We need a new business culture. I want to make a complaint. Having been in hospital many times the least thing you get is decent sleep, which provides the best healing! Noise, shift transitions for nurses, and early morning procedures are all unsettling. And if you stand up they pinch your bed for someone else!

Apart from individual effects, there is also an economic penalty from lack of sleep as it can lead to a loss of productivity. It has been calculated by the global policy think tank of the Rand Corporation that insufficient sleep typically robs nations of about 2% of their GDP through lost productivity. In New Zealand, that was about $4 billion each year. Not only that, lack of sleep causes a 13% higher risk of mortality among workers. It can also make us more prone to accidents. About 15-25% of all fatal driving accidents are caused by sleepiness.

Professor Gander also cited an early 2000s study in New Zealand that found that injury accidents on Auckland roads could be reduced by an astonishing 19% if people avoided driving when they felt sleepy and if they'd had less than five hours' sleep in the previous 24 hours (or between 2am and 5am when the physiological sleep drive peaks).

The situation is no different overseas. Giving just one example from the US, the authors Ford, Cunningham, and Croft (2015) found that 29.2% of adults reported sleeping no more that 6 hours per night and 8.6% reported sleeping at least 9 hours per night. The Centers for Disease Control and Prevention estimated that as many as 70 million Americans have a sleep disorder, and described the situation as a public health epidemic. For further data on the US see https://www.sleepadvisor.org/sleep-statistics/. Walker (2018:243) in referring to his book on sleep said:

> It is probable that that two out of three people reading this book will have difficulty falling or staying asleep at least one night every week.

1.4 WHY DO WE SLEEP?

Dr Nierenberg (2016) asked this very question. He said we are not 100% certain why we sleep, but pointed out what happens when we don't get enough sleep. We can become grumpy, impulsive, and make wrong decisions. Learning, memory, and problem solving can be improved with deep sleep, and it also leads to learning new skills more quickly. That is why cramming the night before an exam doesn't usually pay off. Without enough sleep, you won't retain the new information or skills you learned. Poor sleep can make it more difficult for a person to deal with depression, anxiety, and any other psychological problems that may be present. It is also more difficult to deal with emotional information, which can hurt human relationships. Who wants to live or be with a grumpy person as over-tiredness can prevent thinking before speaking and acting? As already noted above, sleep loss can cause a number health issues, compromising health and safety, productivity, and quality of life. All major organs and our brain are improved by sleep and are negatively affected when we don't get enough sleep.

1.4.1 Brain Cleans Itself

A key aspect of sleep is that the brain cleans itself with fluid when we sleep, with the pulsing, washing mechanism washing away that sticky, toxic, amyloid protein that leads to Alzheimer's disease. Research published in the journal Science found that the brain's cleaning activities increased 10-fold during sleep, helping to remove the day's toxic clutter (NZ Herald, October, 2013). It does it by expanding channels between neurons (brain cells) that allow an influx of cerebrospinal fluid (like detergent!). Also it does it twice as fast when we are sleeping as when awake. In fact the clean-up process is so energy-intensive that it would hinder our thinking if done when we were awake. Dr Nedergaard of University of Rochester Medical Centre in New York said:

> The brain has to choose between being awake and aware of asleep and cleaning up.

He also said:

> You can think of it like having a house party. You can either entertain the guests or clean up the house, but you can't really do both at the same time.

Therefore if you don't have sufficient sleep, the rubbish is going to build up, with serious effects; a bit like an overflowing rubbish bin.

A key part to adequate sleep is the biological clock, which we now discuss.

1.5   THE BIOLOGICAL CLOCK

I have a bedside clock that tends to run a little slow so I have to adjust it occasionally. We all have a biological clock that needs to be adjusted from time to time such as when we travel overseas or go through the process of daylight saving when we gain or lose an hour. All human beings, and most living organisms, are dependent on a circadian rhythm which has been shown to be independent of light. The word 'circadian' comes from the Latin 'circa' which means 'approximately' and 'diem' meaning 'a day', where 'approximately' means being slightly longer than 24 hours. However, daylight is not the only clock setter as there are other biological processes that can help stabilise to a strict 24 hour cycle. These other circadian rhythms are internal cycles that affect the pace of our biological processes such as our preferred times for eating and drinking, our core body temperature, our metabolic rate, and the release of numerous hormones.

We know from scientific studies that we need to keep our circadian rhythm in step with daylight hours seeing that it influences everything from temperature regulation to hormone release and even digestion. When we have an irregular circadian rhythm we can end up with a number of health problems including mental and psychological problems. People with mood disorders such as depression, schizophrenia, seasonal affective disorder (SAD), and bipolar disease have been shown to have disrupted circadian rhythms. Our ability to effectively respond to stress is also impacted by our biological clocks. Various systems that regulate stress, such as the hypothalamus-pituitary-adrenal axis (did you know you had one of these) and the autonomic nervous system receive strong circadian input.

Before there was electricity, the circadian rhythm was determined by natural light so we tended to go to sleep at sunset and wake up at sunrise. However, the invention of artificial light changed all that, especially with the the increased use of light-emitting electronic devices. In fact one study showed that melatonin, the "go to sleep hormone", was reduced by as much as 50 percent in those who read using electronic devices.

The circadian clock receives light information exclusively from a special type of neuron (also known as a neurone or nerve cell) in the eye and is predominantly influenced by blue light, which has a short wave length. The clock can be delayed through exposure to such short wavelengths in the evening, including from domestic lighting, and in particular from computer, cell phone, and TV screens. This exposure makes it harder to fall asleep and wake in the morning, and impedes our attention. Exposure to blue light from the sky is greatest around midday when you want to be well awake.

The history of the biological clock goes back several centuries. For example, French astronomer Jean Jacques d'Ortuous de Mairan in 1729 observed the opening and closing of plants in response to what appeared to be the sunlight. However, by putting plants in a darkened environment he found that the opening and closing of the leaves continued despite the lack of sunlight. He therefore concluded that there must be an internal clock regulating biological rhythms of living organisms.

1.5.1   Role of Biological Clock

Our clock timing system consists of genes and proteins that work together through a feedback loop to keep our biological clocks staying in tune with our environment. When the internal clock genes are activated, they trigger the production of proteins that build up and reach a point when the genes are signalled to switch off. As the proteins degrade, the genes switch on again. This recurring cycle takes approximately 24 hours in a human body.

Technically, our internal clock is located in our brain's hypothalamus in an area called the suprachiasmatic nucleus (SCN). This nucleus is situated close to the area of the brain where the fibre optic bunch of nerve fibres cross, enabling it to regulate itself on a 24-hour cycle using cues from the sunlight. As there have been other internal clock experiments like those with fruit flies, which also are affected by circadian rhythms, it has been suggested that the SCN is a master regulator of all the internal clocks. We are finding that nearly every function our body is tied to our biological clocks. For example, the sleep hormone melatonin is produced in the pineal gland and is responsible for our body's daily cycle. As daylight decreases there is less light into the SCN causing an increase of melatonin production, and this tells our body to go into sleep mode. Melatonin is discussed in more detail later.

Daylight is not the only thing that the the body can use for resetting the biological clock as the brain can also use external cues such as food, exercise, and temperature changes, if they are regular.

Sleep pressure

Another factor affecting sleep is so-called 'sleep pressure'. It is caused by a chemical called adenosine that builds up in the brain throughout the day and makes us feel more sleepy. Adenosine levels peak in people after 12–16 hours of being awake. We can "mute the signal" of adenosine using caffeine, which competes with adenosine for receptors in the brain. Sleep degrades and removes the adenosine, so naps (discussed in section 3.1) reduce sleep pressure, and eight hours will clear it out. The two systems, the circadian wake drive and the sleep drive, actually work independently, though they are usually aligned.

Hormones affected

I have already mentioned that some hormones are affected by our circadian rhythm. For example, ghrelin and leptin (not gremlin and leprechaun) are responsible for promoting and suppressing hunger, respectively, and they follow a rhythmic cycle as well. It has been found that sleep deprivation increases levels of ghrelin and decreases the levels of leptin, causing individuals to eat more when tired. Have you noticed this? Leptin is also important in bone formation so that sleep strengthens bone structure. Getting sufficient sleep helps the body process glucose so that lack of sleep can lead to an increased risk of diabetes. The brain consumes up to two thirds of the circulating glucose so that major changes in brain activity such as those associated with sleep-wake and wake-sleep transitions are going to impact glucose metabolism (Morselli, Guyon, and Spiegeli, 2012). Also lack of sleep increases blood pressure and makes the body more exposed to inflammation, thus increasing heart disease risks.

When sleeping, the body self-repairs by producing hormones that repair damaged tissues. Therefore, cutting back on sleep can for example reduce skin thickening and healing. It can also reduce both male and female fertility because it lowers the amount of reproductive hormones the body produces. For example, it lowers testosterone levels and sperm counts in men, and reduces follicular-releasing hormones in women. Also, for women, it can interfere with menstrual cycles and increases the risk of miscarriage in pregnancy.

Cortisol, the so-called stress hormone involved with our fight or flight response, is responsible for helping to regulate the stress response. In a healthy person we find that its level in the blood tends to rise dramatically as the night progresses starting about 2-3 hour after sleep onset, reaching its maximum around sunrise. It then falls slowly during the day down to its lowest level late in the evening. Studies have shown that even slight sleep disturbances result in elevated cortisol levels, which in turn causes wakefulness. Finally, the production of serotonin, the feel good hormone, is directly related to sunlight exposure. It increases during the time of day when there is more light. Serotonin is also a building block for melatonin.

1.6 HOW MUCH SLEEP?

An important question is: "How much sleep do we need?" The answer is: "Usually more than we think," though we are not very good at gauging how much sleep we actually get. Women usually need a little more sleep than men. There is a condition called sleep-state misperception (paradoxical insomnia) when people report having slept badly during the night when in fact sleep monitoring has shown they have slept much better than what they believe, and in fact may have had a very good sleep. Psychological help is available for this problem.

The gold standard for sleep in the past has been eight hours a night of solid, uninterrupted sleep, but there has been some controversy about this. Many people know they do not need eight hours sleep and cannot sleep eight hours even if they try. We have to be careful how we set standards as we do not want to pressure people into taking sleeping pills. A study by Kripke, Langer, et al. (2011) confirmed that using wrist actigraphy (section 1.13) the graph of mortality risk versus hours of of sleep was U-shaped, that is the graph of mortality versus amount of sleep falls, then levels out, and then rises like a U. This means that both short sleep and long sleep are associated with excess mortality. In other words too little or too much sleep can be detrimental. An earlier follow-up study by Hublin, Markku, et al. (2007) using 21,268 twins found that those sleeping less that 7 hours and those greater than 8 hours had a higher mortality than those sleeping 7-8 hours. This was supported by a large review and meta-analysis incorporating 1.38 million people by Cappuccio, D'Elia, et al. (2010). It was also supported by a similar review and meta-analysis by Gallicchio and Kalesan (2009) who used an upper criterion of greater than nine hours rather than eight hours.

Walker (2018:140), writing from thirty years of intensive sleep research, said that after 16 hours of being awake the brain begins to fail so that we need more than seven hours of sleep each night to maintain cognitive performance. Clearly it may help if we spend 8 hours in bed so that it gives us opportunity for further sleep, even if it does not happen for all that time. If we only have six hours in bed at night the amount of sleep time will be even less. Also the adenosine (sleep pressure) that has accumulated carries on to the next night and can therefore continues to accumulate, causing chronic tiredness. Although there is considerable individual variation, a range of between 7 and 9 hours a night is generally regarded as an acceptable range for adults as we are all different and one hat does not fit all heads. Genetics can also play an important part. The US National Sleep Foundation has the following recommendations for healthy individuals from a large review panel (Hirshkowitz, Whiton, et al., 2015):

Older adults (65+): 7–8 hours.

Young Adults and Adults (18–64 years): 7–9 hours.

Teenagers (14–17 years): 8–10 hours.

School children (6–13 years): 9–11 hours.

Preschoolers (3–5 years): 10–13 hours.

Toddlers (1–2 years): 11–14 hours.

Infants (4–11 months): 12–15 hours.

Newborns (0–3 months): 14–17 hours.

The authors also give lower levels that may be appropriate on occasion and inadequate levels to be avoided.

1.7 GETTING ENOUGH SLEEP?

We may not be getting enough sleep if we always need an alarm clock to wake us up, we habitually sleep late on weekends, we could drop off to sleep mid morning and need caffeine to get going, and we fall asleep during meetings, watching TV, and reading. One suggested test is to set an alarm for 15 minutes and if we fall asleep in that time we have a problem. We eventually pay for a lack of sleep if we draw too much on our sleep bank. Deep sleep is a very important part of the sleep cycle (see chapter 2) as it is restorative. Stress, anxiety and depression can affect the sleeping pattern. It is the quality of our sleep not the quantity that is important. Also you cannot catch up on quality sleep just once or twice a week, say on the weekend with a sleep "binge". If an average person gets less than six hours of good sleep each night, they are sleep deprived. Sleep deprivation can mess up our emotions with that part of the brain called the amygdala causing over-reacting and emotional swings. Been touchy lately?

There are two systems in our brain that regulate both sleep and wakefulness; a wakefulness system that dominates during the day and keeps us awake, and a sleep system that dominates at night (Jacobs, 1999:20). However, the wakefulness system is always "on guard" even in our deepest sleep so that we are never completely oblivious to the outside world. A person with a weak sleep system or an over-strong wakefulness system may be more vulnerable to sleep problems.

1.7.1 The Elderly

One myth is that sleep needs decrease with age. This is not true. Older people need about the same amount of sleep as younger people, but they are not so good at achieving it. They will often only have one period of deep sleep during the night, usually in the first 3 or 4 hours, after which they wake more easily. They also take longer to fall asleep, with the amount and length of their waking points during the night increasing with age, and the time spent in deep sleep decreasing. There is also a tendency to dream less as people get older. Retirement can also trigger sleep problems as a person's job gives them their internal clock, and sleep can suffer without a daily routine. Being in my 80's I find these situations to be the case.

The quality of our dream (REM) sleep (see chapter 2) often affects how we think, feel, and act during the day. Deep sleep helps to produce growth hormone that restores energy, immunity, healing, weight loss, memory improvement, and lowered blood pressure and pulse. One way to find out how much sleep we need is to try adding half an hour at a time (about a week apart) until there is no improvement on waking; a good time to experiment is when on holiday. The main requirement of sleep is that we get both deep sleep and dream sleep, that is quality sleep. Even just one night of insufficient sleep can have a major affect next day.

Unfortunately insomnia becomes more common as we age, as sleep becomes less restful and lighter, particularly with environmental changes (e.g., noise, rise in temperature) being more likely to wake us up. As already indicated above, deep sleep deteriorates as we age, and this is linked to a decline in memory. Some age factors affecting sleep are a reduction in melatonin production and growth hormone, changes in body temperature, an increase in bladder problems, less physically or socially active, and sometimes less exposure to natural light. Also a person's internal clock often advances, so they get tired earlier in the evening and wake up earlier in the morning.

Then of course there are health changes and medications that can interfere with sleep. Walker (2018:96-97) makes an important point that with aging health deterioration we usually concentrate on health issues and ignore the sleep effect and medical help for it, other than sleeping tablets. Also, as we age, our sleep becomes more fragmented so that we wake up more frequently during the night, and the proportion of the bedtime we are asleep, called sleep efficiency, goes down. Unfortunately the parts of the brain that promote deep sleep break down the earliest and most severely as we age (Walker, 2018:102). Furthermore, the strength of the circadian rhythm and the amount of nighttime melatonin released decrease as we get older. We need to avoid early evening naps as they deplete the sleep pressure causing wakefulness later, which is compounded by the shift to early rising.

1.8 EFFECTS OF SLEEP DEPRIVATION

I have mentioned above the effects of sleep deprivation on health. Walker (2018:3–5) said that routinely sleeping less than six or seven hours a night demolishes our immune system (by reducing the production of cytokines that target infection and inflammation), more than doubles the risk of cancer, and, as mentioned above, is a key lifestyle factor in determining whether or not we develop Alzheimer's disease. He says:

> the shorter your sleep, the shorter your life span.

and

> sleep is the single most effective thing we can do to reset our brain and body health each day.

Former British Prime Minister Margaret Thatcher said she needed only four hours' sleep at night but later developed dementia; perhaps a connection. Walker (2018) mentioned that under-sleeping increases the likelihood of having furred and brittle arteries, laying us open to the risk of heart attacks and strokes. Even moderate reductions of sleep for a week can disrupt blood-sugar levels so severely that a person can be classified as pre-diabetic.

Research on the sleeping habits of 3,019 patients over the age of 45 found that those who slept less than six hours were found twice as likely to have a stroke or heart attack, and over 1.6 times more likely to develop congestive heart failure. A study called Whitehall 2 examined the sleeping habits of over 10,000 British government employees. They found that those employees who slept the least doubled their risk of death.

Lack of sleep also affects our memory. Recent research carried out in the USA and France showed that the body uses sleep time to transfer information to the brain. Cutting back on sleep deprives the body of these opportunities to boost memory functioning. Also, sleep deprivation can mess up our emotions, with that part of the brain called the amygdala over-reacting and causing emotional swings. Been touchy lately?

Having focused on negative aspects of sleep deprivation, let us now sum up some positive aspects of having adequate sleep. According to an article from the NZ Listener magazine, adequate sleep helps you to live longer, boosts your memory and creativity, keeps you slim and makes you better looking (must get some more sleep). It also helps to guard you from cancer and dementia, lower your risk of heart attacks, stroke and diabetes, and keeps away colds and the flu. You'll even feel happier, less depressed, and less anxious. Also good sleep improves physical performance. Sleep before a game not only helps a person to perform better but also helps faster recovery after the hard work has been done, says Walker (2018), who often speaks to professional sports teams about the role of sleep. A chronic lack of sleep accurately predicts a massively higher risk of injury.

1.8.1 Micro Sleep

One of the dangers of insufficient sleep is that you can have a micro sleep lasting just even a couple of seconds when you lose complete contact with the outside world. In a car this can mean a major accident and loss of life. If you are feeling sleepy when driving you need to pull over and have a rest. This happened to me a long time ago when driving a camper-van with my two young sons through a lot of rain. I was probably hypnotised by the windscreen wipers and was suffering from less sleep the previous night in the van. I suddenly found myself off the road and driving on a green strip parallel to the road with trees rapidly coming up. I could not brake as water was spraying from the waterlogged ground so I had to somehow steer back on the road at a wobbly high speed. Normally there is a ditch alongside the road so I was grateful there wasn't one just at that time. I pulled over for a rest. I had learnt my lesson. One of the problems is when you are sleep deprived you may not realise it.

1.8.2   Our Chronotype

An important aspect of sleep is that we are not all the same, and we need to heed our chronotype, that is whether we are a morning person (a "lark") or an evening person (an "owl"), and plan our sleep accordingly. Otherwise our various cycles such as food intake, sleep-wake, and metabolic cycles may not work together, but can get out of sync and can, for example, cause a variety of problems and accelerate aging. According to Walker (2018:20), about 40% are "morning types", 30% are "evening types", and the balance of 30% in between; the type is largely determined by genetics. Larks like to wake up earlier, go to bed earlier, and function better in the morning, while owls like to wake up later, go to bed later, and function better at night. One problem is that people often have to leave for work or start work very early, thus penalising the owls and perhaps forcing them to work at both ends of the day. Such differences need to be taken into account in designing work schedules. The current trend of working from home would help this situation.

1.9   CAFFEINE AND ALCOHOL

Some strategies and hints for improving sleep are summarised in chapter 3 and the Appendix A.1. I mention a few here about things to avoid food-wise. Caffeine can be a sleep disrupter. It is found, for example, in energy drinks, tea, coffee, ice cream, dark chocolate, and some medications. Having a half-life of six hours means that half the caffeine is still in our system 6 hours later and a quarter 12 hours later, which can disturb sleep. Technically, caffeine interferes with the sleep pressure of adenosine in our brains to make us more alert. This means we have to decide at what time of the day we stop caffeine intake. For those with a sleep problem this may mean stopping caffeine intake after the morning break or early in the afternoon. Once the caffeine is metabolised by the liver, there is a "crash" when the build up of sleep pressure from the adenosine that was previously overridden by the caffeine causes an attack of over-sleepiness. This will not help if we are trying to stay awake longer. However, caffeine affects everyone differently and some people can tolerate black tea or coffee better than others because of certain genes speeding up the liver breakdown of the caffeine. Also, the older we are the longer it takes to get rid of the caffeine. It should be noted that so called decaffeinated coffee is not caffeine free as it can contain 15% or more of that in regular coffee. Irrespective of our sleepiness or wakefulness, the twenty-four hour circadian rhythm marches on with its rising and falling according to the time of night or day it is. It is oblivious to our lack of sleep.

Another no-no before sleep is drinking alcohol just before bedtime. According to sleep specialist Dr Michael Breus, around 20 percent of adult Americans use alcohol to help them fall asleep. In fact many people believe that a glass or two at night helps them sleep better. Unfortunately this is not true and alcohol actually disturbs your sleep. It may help a person initially to drop off to sleep but it causes wakefulness and broken and disturbed sleep later. In fact just two standard drinks can affect sleep in multiple ways. On average, two standard drinks take two hours to metabolise. Walker (2018:82) said that alcohol is one of the most suppressors of REM (dream) sleep that we know of. Alcohol should be totally avoided if a woman wishes to become pregnant or is pregnant, as no amount of alcohol is safe for such a person, nor for anyone else (Seber and Woodfield, 2020).

What happens with alcohol is that we become relaxed because alcohol affects the prefrontal cortex area of our brain first, the impulse-control part (dancing on the table time), and then it begins to sedate other parts as well. However, Walker says,

> The electrical brainwave state you enter via alcohol is not that of natural sleep. Rather, it is akin to a light form of anaesthesia.

You wake up later and have difficulty in getting back to sleep. In fact alcohol is converted to acetaldehyde (a carcinogen) by the liver (Seber and Woodfield, 2020). Because of these factors, Walker said that

> alcohol is one of the most powerful suppressors of REM sleep that we know of.

and Rapid Eye Movement (REM) sleep is essential for good health. Because of the relaxing quality of alcohol, drinking before bed can relax the muscles around the mouth and throat, thus increasing the risk of snoring. We also urinate more, thus disrupting sleep. REM sleep and further details are given later in chapter 2 on sleep cycles.

1.10   SHIFT WORKERS

A tremendous amount of research surrounds the health of shift workers, such as nurses and doctors who work nights in a hospital, and airline pilots. Gander, O'Keefe, et al. (2019) said that

> Workplace fatigue is now recognised as a physiologically-based state of impaired performance caused by four main factors: (1) sleep loss (acute

and chronic); (2) extended time awake (more than about 16 h); (3) working and sleeping at sub-optimal times in the circadian body clock cycle; and (4) physical and mental workload.

The problem is that the circadian body clock that regulates sleep timing and quality very rarely adapts fully to shift work. Apparently only a small percentage percent of people adapt physiologically to night shifts, especially for those who switch to a normal weekend sleep schedule. This means that nurses, for example, who are fatigued from shift work and extended hours can compromise patient care and increase the risk of clinical error. Unfortunately shift work, and particularly night work, can also have long-term negative effects on nurses' health. In general, working nights for anyone has been linked with increased rates of heart disease, cancer, diabetes, obesity, and depression, just to name a few. Studies have shown that individuals who get insufficient sleep are also impacted by the same health problems that face shift workers. Proper protocols need to be in place to protect shift workers such as the National Code of Practice (2019).

There are ways of getting adequate sleep while doing shift work. To begin with, the key is to adjust the body temperature cycle as soon as possible, which means endeavouring to adjust in advance when there is a change in shift time coming up. One can make use of bright light or conversely avoiding it by wearing sunglasses, which are strategies that can be used to shift the temperature cycle. If you are a shift worker and have difficulty sleeping during the day, the chances are that you also have difficulty staying awake at work. Here are some tips for staying alert on the job from SleepFoundation.org:

- Avoid long commutes and extended hours.

- Take short nap breaks throughout the shift.

- Work with others to help keep you alert.

- Try to be active during breaks (e.g., take a walk, shoot hoops in the parking lot, or even exercise).

- Drink a caffeinated beverage (coffee, tea, colas) to help maintain alertness during the shift.

- Don't leave the most tedious or boring tasks to the end of your shift when you are apt to feel the drowsiest. Night shift workers are most sleepy around 4-5 a.m.

- Exchange ideas with your colleagues on ways to cope with the problems of shift work. Set up a support group at work so that you can discuss these issues and learn from each other.

Also from SleepFoundation.org we have following tips for sleeping during the day.

- Wear dark glasses to block out the sunlight on your way home.
- Keep to the same bedtime and wake time schedule, even on weekends.
- Eliminate noise and light from your sleep environment (use eye masks and ear plugs if necessary).
- Avoid caffeinated beverages, foods, and alcohol close to bedtime.

Some of the above apply to anyone with sleep difficulties (Appendix A.1).

1.11 DRIVING

Closely related to the previous topic is long distance and/or night driving. In addition to those who do it for a living, we all probably have to face this at some time in our lives. The NZ Transport Agency has the following fatigue warning signs:

- Yawning (usually one of the first symptoms).
- Your head starts nodding.
- Restlessness. Changing your position frequently (unless you are genuinely uncomfortable).
- Drowsiness. Your head starts nodding.
- You have trouble keeping your eyes open. Blinking frequently. Rubbing your eyes and finding it difficult to focus.
- Braking too late.
- Lack of concentration (your mind wanders and you realise that you have just driven the last 5km and do not remember a thing about it).
- Difficulty staying in your lane and drifting from side to side.
- Feeling irritable.

The Agency also has the following recommendations when driving in general to avoid nodding off at the wheel:

- Get enough sleep regularly.

- Snack lightly, choosing light fresh food. Avoid fatty, sugary or carbohydrate-filled options.

- Take a break from driving at least every two hours.

- Power nap for no more that 20 minutes for best effect.

- Drive during times when usually awake. Take care after a meal.

- Drinking water helps keep one alert.

- Keep a check on any medication as some can cause drowsiness..

- Share the driving if possible.

- Avoid alcohol.

Coffee, fresh air, and music will help fatigue short term.

1.12 SLEEP AND AGE GROUPS

Although we are all different, there are some common factors about sleep for each age group. During adolescence the circadian rhythm tends to be later than that for adults with a tendency to go to bed later and get up later. This means that for some it may be natural to not be able to fall asleep before 11:00 pm. In addition, adolescents need more sleep. This has led some countries to changing the school starting time to a later time as children are then more awake. There is evidence that children who sleep longer tend to do better academically. Under-sleep is not going to help a child and this has been happening more in recent times. Unfortunately most parents don't realise this. There is also the question of a connection between lack of sleep and ADHD (Attention Deficit Hyperactivity Disorder). It is therefore important not to label such sleep-in behaviour as laziness as teenagers are wired that way. The circadian rhythm does shift to a later period as they get older and head towards adulthood.

Stanley (2018) writes about sleep and age as follows. In one's 20s a person is inclined to burn the candle at both ends, and seems to be able to get away with it. Also those under about 27 years tend to be night owls, which can be a problem when they enter the work force.

In one's 30s, work, financial stress, and raising a family all kick in. For women, pregnancy can bring insomnia and waking throughout the night. As many as one in four pregnant women are affected by restless legs syndrome (Appendix A.4.1). Low iron is a common trigger and supplements can treat it. A disturbed night's sleep leaves you feeling as bad as an extremely short sleep. A 2014 study by Tel Aviv University found that women who slept for eight hours, but were woken four times, were as groggy and tired as women who had slept for just four hours. Stanley says

> Once a child gets past feeding, my advice is to take turns on night time duties rather than splitting them in the same night.

and

> If you can, agree in advance who's going to get up if a child wakes, while the other person sleeps through - with ear plugs in if needs be - and take turns that way.

In one's 40s Walker (2018:96) notes that there is a

> palpable reduction in the electrical quantity and quality of that deep NREM sleep.

There are fewer hours of such sleep, and the brain waves accompanying that sleep become smaller, less powerful, and fewer in number. In the mid- and late forties one loses 60 to 70 percent of the deep sleep experienced as a young teenager. This loss increases with age.

For those in their 50's it is common for sleep to be disturbed because of having to get up to go to the toilet. Women going through the menopause between the ages of 40 and 59 are more likely than both post- and pre-menopausal women to sleep for less than seven hours a night, according to US research. Hot flushes are likely to be the biggest problem, as to fall asleep you need to lose one degree of body heat. This means anything that raises body temperature at night should avoided.

For the 60's the aging effect kicks in, as previously mentioned in section 1.7.1. . Older men, for example, may have REM (dream) sleep behaviour disorders such as starting to act out their dreams at night, where normally the brain would keep them paralysed.

In the 70's and older, insomnia is very common. Part of the reason is that less time is spent in REM sleep, which is also restorative sleep, leading to feeling more tired and less refreshed from sleep. In fact Walker (2018) says that by seventy, one has lost 80 to 90 percent of youthful deep sleep.

As mentioned above, as we get older our body clock tends to shift forward pushing a person to get up and go to bed much earlier (the reverse of a teenager). Getting more natural light, especially in the afternoon and early evening, may help to delay the onset of melatonin so that spending a lot of time indoors is not helpful.

1.13   METHODS OF STUDYING SLEEP

We can, of course, keep track of how much we sleep ourselves, though this is not easy as it is subjective and keeping track can interfere with our sleep duration because of clock watching. One method that has been used since the early 1970's is polysomnography (PSG) or sleep study, which is usually an overnight series of tests to evaluate sleeping. For example, an EEG monitors one's brain activity to identify sleep cycles and disturbances, an EOG monitors eye movement, an EMG monitors muscle activity, and an ECG monitors heart rhythm. A sleep specialist can then use this information as well as, for example, breathing and oxygen levels to find out whether a person has a sleep disorder. It is not recommended for the evaluation of insomnia unless there is suspected underlying sleep apnea, paradoxical insomnia, or parasomnia.

Another method is to use an actigraph, a device generally placed on the wrist to record movement that is relayed to a computer for analysis. It is based on the idea that there is less movement when asleep than when awake. The method has the advantage that it can conveniently record continuously for 24-hours a day for days, weeks or even longer, and can be used at home, providing a cheaper option and eliminating laboratory effects. It has been used to monitor insomnia, circadian sleep/wake disturbances, and periodic limb movement disorder, and is particularly useful in measuring night-to-night changes in sleep patterns. Ancoli-Israel, Cole et al. (2003) gave a review of the method and its shortcomings, and compared it with other study methods such as the traditional gold standard PSG above.

SLEEP STAGES

2.1 THE SLEEP CYCLE

Research has shown that every 90 minutes or longer we go through a pattern of non-dream sleep (NREM or non-rapid eye movement sleep) followed by a short period of dream sleep (REM or rapid eye movement sleep). The NREM sleep consist of four stages 1–4 that cycle through 1,2,3,4,3,2. Stages 1 and 2 are essentially light sleep and 3 and 4 are deep sleep, depending on the brain waves. When we go to bed we find that after about 15 or so minutes of relaxation we reach a stage of semiconsciousness that is neither waking nor sleeping (stage 1) for a few minutes as slowing alpha waves prepare us for sleep. We then suddenly fall into a light sleep (stage 2) when eye movement stops. Brain waves slow down with occasional bursts of activity called sleep spindles (short and powerful bursts of electrical activity in the brain), discussed further below. Breathing, heart rate, metabolic rate, and body temperature continue to drop as we prepare for deeper sleep. After about thirty to forty-five minutes in stage 2 we go into the deeper stages

3 and finally 4 where we enjoy long, slow-wave sleep. We then go back through stages 3 and 2, and enter dream sleep. Here breathing becomes shallow, rapid and irregular in response to dreaming, and eyes move rapidly and limb muscles are temporarily paralysed. As the night progresses, the deeper stages of sleep gets shorter and the REM stage gets longer. This pattern appears to help the brain find the ideal balance between keeping in our memory what's old but useful and leaving sufficient room for the new. (I find that for every new item added, two drop out!)

As we go through these cycles, it is normal to have short periods of wakefulness of 1 or 2 minutes between cycles (especially with older people). We are not usually aware of them unless we are anxious or disturbed. The short periods of being awake feel much longer than they really are so we may feel that we are not sleeping as much as we actually are. We therefore don't need to feel anxious about these waking periods. The NREM sleep helps transfer and consolidate newly learned information into long-term memory and weeds out unnecessary neural connections, says Walker (2018), while dreaming REM sleep strengthens those connections. Also some memories lost soon after learning can be regained after sleep.

This memory improvement through sleep is true for all age groups, and even for some primates. NREM sleep, particularly when packed with sleep spindles mentioned above, also helps cement motor skills such as riding a bike, playing sport, or playing the piano. Walker (2018:124-125) noted that, with regard to piano playing and skill learning in general, the brain continues to improve those memories through sleep without further practice. He said:

> It is practice followed by a night of sleep that leads to perfection.

As a musician I was surprised at this, and it has encouraged me to get back into music again. With regard to sport and athletics, regular sleep and even naps can improve performance, reduce injury risk, and promote recovery after an injury. It also helps with stroke recovery. Unfortunately there is the temptation to cut short these last special hours of sleep to get the day going early, which is clearly not a good idea.

Deep sleep (slow wave or delta sleep) is particularly important as physical energy is restored, memory strongly improved, and learning capacity increased. It is also the stage most associated with weird behaviours such as sleep-walking and sleep-talking. The brain uses this sleep stage to replay the activities from the day. It is why cramming the night before an exam does not usually pay off, as without enough sleep you won't retain the new information or previously learned skills on waking. Each sleep stage, consisting of light NREM sleep, deep NREM sleep, and REM sleep, provides a different positive benefit to our brains at different times of the night, so all the stages are needed. For example, our emotional intelligence depends on getting our quota of REM sleep, as it fine-tunes the emotional circuits of the brain.

Sleep Spindles

Although I have already mentioned the key role of sleep spindles, I wish to say a bit more about them. Walker (2018:110) said that the memory improvement that comes with the spindles refers to (his italics)

> the *change* in learning from before relative to after sleep, which is to say the 'replenishment' of learning ability, that spindles predicted.

In other words, the sleep does not take you above your natural ability but helps it to work best with what you have. The more spindles generated the better as far as the brain's capacity to re-store learning and make room for new memories, with previous learning transferred to a more permanent and stable residence in longterm memory. This is where napping can help memory con-solidation, provided it contains enough NREM sleep. The more sleep spindles obtained during a nap, and these can occur dur-ing both the light and deep stages of NREM sleep, the greater the restoration of learning capacity when waking. Unfortunately the elderly (60 to 80 years) are unable to generate the spindles to the same degree as young healthy adults, but suffer a 40 percent deficit. (Now I know why I can't find my glasses or forget things.)

2.2   BODY TEMPERATURE AND LIGHT

Body temperature is a key to how we sleep. It goes through a daily cycle (circadian rhythm) closely linked to our activity levels and sleep pattern (Jacobs (1999:19) reaching its maximum around 6 p.m. and then steadily dropping over the following hours later until bedtime. Our temperature then declines more rapidly to its minimum around 4.00 a.m. and then begins to increase just before sunrise. It continues to increase until lunch time and then drops somewhat after lunch before increasing until about 6 p.m. again. The higher temperatures are linked to activity and alertness, and lower temperatures to sleepiness, irrespective of how we slept the night before. Sleep and body temperature are directly influenced by the daily cycles of sunlight and darkness and their effect on the neurotransmitter melatonin in the brain. Those with insomnia tend to have higher day and night body temperatures.

When the amount of light entering our eyes goes up, melatonin levels go down and our body temperature goes up, and all vice versa. When an environment has more light, the brain assumes it is daytime and produces less melatonin. Darkness encourages melatonin production because the brain interprets this as night. In general, the rise in melatonin begins between 8 p.m. and 10 p.m., peaks between 2 a.m and 4 a.m., then declines gradually over the morning.

With body temperature, different body temperature cycles explain why some people function best in the morning, while others function better in the evening. Since our sleep is related to our body temperature it is important that we get up the same time every morning to start our body-temperature rhythm. If we sleep in, say for more than an hour, we delay the rise in our body temperature in the morning, delay the fall at night, and thus upset our temperature cycle. For example, sleeping in on Sunday morning may therefore affect our sleep on Sunday night, especially if we try to go to bed earlier to prepare for the week ahead. It would then be better to go to bed later.

It should be noted that red light, being of relatively low intensity, can help with melatonin production, while blue light is of higher intensity and can inhibit the beneficial effects of melatonin. In addition to sunlight, which has blue light, we find that blue light from televisions, computer screens, and cell phones causes a decrease in melatonin production, making it harder to fall asleep. Experts recommend staying off screens from at least half an hour to as much as two hours before bedtime, or else use special glasses blocking blue light after sunset. Some devices have a blocking system built in.

Researchers found that new memories form during slow-wave sleep. You may know it as delta sleep. Its a deep stage of sleep that is hard to wake up from. Not surprisingly, this is also the stage most associated with weird behaviours like sleep-walking and sleep-talking. The brain uses this sleep stage to replay the activities from the day. Spending time in this stage may also increase a person's capacity for learning.

Sleep Efficiency

What is important is one's sleep efficiency mentioned briefly in chapter 1, which refers to the percentage of time spent in bed that a person is asleep. Good sleepers may have an efficiency of at least 90% (i.e. asleep for at least 90% of the time in bed) while a poor sleeper might only manage 65%. For the former group bed becomes associated with sleep, while for the latter bed can become associated with wakefulness. The key is to go to bed later but get up the same time every morning to achieve the required efficiency of at least 90%. One recommendation is to first find one's sleep efficiency over say 5 days. If it increases to greater than 90%, the sleeper is allowed 15 minutes of additional time in bed by going to bed earlier. If sleep efficiency decreases to below 85%, then their time in bed is further curtailed by a similar amount. Initially it may mean going to bed very late to get sleepy enough. Staying awake long enough may be a problem so that some mild activity might be needed earlier on in the evening. Summing up, once sleep efficiency is at least 85% for two weeks, the time in bed can be increased by 15 minutes each week while maintaining the 85%. This method is referred to as sleep restriction therapy. By keeping one awake longer a strong sleep pressure can be built up.

2.3   DREAMS

Dreams have always been a subject of speculation and debate without really understanding why we have them. However, with the advent of brain imaging techniques such as MRI (magnetic imaging resonance) in the 21st century enabling scientists to obtain three dimensional images of brain activity during REM sleep, we are now a step closer in our understanding of dreaming. What is interesting is that when dreaming the logical part of our brain controlling rational thought is reduced, but there is a letting loose of the visual, emotional, motor, and personal memory regions. No wonder we can have such vivid dreams. One observation is that most dreams are hard to remember. Women recall more dreams than men, and the older one gets the less the dream recall is reported. However, with some conditioning (e.g., by telling ourselves a few times in a row that we will remember our dreams), dreams can be remembered long enough to be written down.

Some people have used dreams to obtain psychological help (see Seber, 2013:39). I believe it is helpful when you have a dream with an ending you do not like is to change the ending when you wake up, putting something positive back into the subconscious. If you happen to sleep in one morning you are likely to dream and perhaps dream for longer time. When people had to stay isolation because of the Ovid 19 virus that affected the whole world, people were more likely to sleep in. It is a good idea for a person to share their dreams with others as it helps to create empathy.

What causes dreams?

Walker (2018:204 and chapter 10), after reviewing the results of an experiment with sleepers, said that

> Dreams are not, therefore, a wholesale replay of our waking lives.

However with REM-sleep dreaming, there is a strong link between dreams at night and the *emotional* concerns of the day, being a metaphor for the latter. For example, a woman may believe that her husband is having an affair, whereas a dream could express a feeling that he has betrayed her. Walker describes dreaming as "nursing our emotional and mental health" and providing "overnight therapy". For example, dreaming shuts off the stress chemical noradrenaline in the brain, so that dreaming about a specific painful experience helps to resolve the emotion attached to the experience. Through dreaming we can express hidden feelings that we find difficult to think or talk about when awake. It also improves emotional acuity where a person can distinguish one emotion from another in other people and be able, for example, to read facial expressions. Dreaming has opened the way to a great deal of creative activity like solving a problem or coming up with a brilliant idea when awakening from dream sleep. It gives strength to the well known phrase "sleep on it."

A variety of things can happen when dreaming such as having nightmares and night terrors, the latter more common with children. Some people grind their teeth (bruxism). Usually these will pass or can be dealt with, though those with post traumatic stress disorder (PTSD) with the recurrence of unpleasant dreams may need psychological help.

We conclude with a few comments on lucid dreaming where you are actually aware that you are dreaming. It is kind of a hybrid state between sleeping and being awake. One possible application of this is in helping people who have nightmares to dream lucidly so that they can consciously wake up. However, its potential for good or harm is still unknown.

STRATEGIES FOR SLEEP

3.1 DURING THE DAY

How we sleep at night tends to relate to what has happened during the day, so, in a sense, we prepare all day for sleep! A good way to start the day is to expose ourselves to bright light/sunlight soon after waking up in the morning to help regulate our biological clock (e.g., open the curtains in summer, turn on the light). Since we know that exercise promotes sleep, some form of exercise needs to be programmed into our day, which is generally not easy if we are busy. Exercise is also a stress reliever and helps with depression.

For most age groups it is better to exercise earlier in the day, which for some means first thing in the morning, or else possibly after work, using a variety of exercise programmes which might include resistance exercises (e.g., weights), exercycling, going for a walk or run, swimming, or going to a gym. Walker (2018:100) suggests two modifications for the elderly who want to reduce shifting to the early-to-rise schedule that goes with aging. First, wear sunglasses if exercising outdoors in the morning, and second, get some sunlight exposure to a part of one's body late afternoon without sunglasses to push back sleep pressure mentioned in chapter 1 and delay the evening release of melatonin. Also vigorous walking is very good for us.

It should be noted that exercising too late at night will tend to wake the body up as one's pulse is elevated. Many years ago I joined a seniors' swimming group in a local indoor pool at night once a week. We swam lengths and had a few races. I eventually had to give it up as I did not sleep too well afterwards as my pulse was elevated at bedtime and I got a bit hot. Our temperature needs to drop by about $1°C$ for sleep. Walker (2018:277) said that a bedroom temperature of around $65°F$ ($18.3°C$) is about right, though it will depend on clothing and bedding. The message is that you sleep better when you are on the cool side.

If you exercise first thing in the morning, it is helpful to eat soon afterwards if not before. During the day one can do a variety of physical activities. For example getting off a bus a bit early and walking the rest of the route to work, using stairs rather than a lift during the day, and standing up while you are on the phone.

It is also a good idea to have some exposure to bright sunlight during the day as it can help with sleep at night and reduce sleep pressure during the day. Sunlight promotes vitamin D3 in our bodies, which is an important vitamin affecting our whole bodies. You might be able to have a walk at lunch time, or at least sit in the sun. Unfortunately many people are stuck in an office and may not even see the sun in winter, going to work in the dark and coming home in the dark.

Stress

It is important to cope with any stress during the day otherwise it tends to come back and haunt one at night. Stress tends to build up during the day and may rise above a certain threshold when it begins to affect one's sleep. It is best to try and reduce any stress throughout the day by having several brief sessions of relaxation exercise. For example, one can use short spells of diaphragm slow breathing and perhaps use some mental exercise as described in section 3.4 below. We can sit in a comfortable chair (the same one each time so it becomes associated with relaxing) and progressively relax our muscles (e.g, telling our limbs that they are getting heavier and heavier). A relaxation technique for tense muscles and a racing mind can produce a brain-wave pattern similar to stage 1 sleep. We also need to avoid any negative self-talk. In any case, if our job requires a lot of sitting we need to take short breaks and do a few sitting and/or standing exercises throughout the day (e.g., every 20 minutes or at least hourly). Anybody else in the work place won't mind. They may end up doing it too.

Naps

What about naps? They are generally regarded as helpful, though some care is needed. For example, there is a universal dip in body temperature after lunch, and Europe is particularly famous for its siesta time. Having a board meeting after lunch will catch people nodding off then waking up with an embarrassing jerk. If you must sleep during the day it is generally best to restrict it to less than 20 minutes early in the afternoon to avoid going into a full sleep cycle, especially deep sleep. US research has found that even catnaps of six minutes can improve learning and memory. However, with severe fatigue, a longer sleep might be needed. If you go into a deep sleep during the day, you won't feel so good for about 10 minutes after you wake up as you suffer from so called "sleep inertia" when you feel you have been hit with a sledge hammer; it can disrupt your nighttime sleep. Dr Leigh Signal from Massey University's Sleep/Wake Research Centre in New Zealand said that 10 minutes' sleep can give benefits for up to two hours; 30 minutes could give up to three hours.

With regard to sleep, infants and children are very different having many short stretches of sleep throughout the day and night with numerous wake-ups, usually accompanied by vocal expressions. It seems that deep NREM sleep is necessary for brain maturation in teenagers.

3.2 PREPARING FOR BED

We now look at a range of activities that will help us with our sleep. We begin with the bedroom.

3.2.1 Environment

We first need to give attention to our bedroom, which means having a good supporting mattress and pillow. Room temperature is important for if the bedroom temperature is too hot it will raise body temperature and affect the sleep cycle. Men are generally more affected by heat than women as they have a higher metabolic rate. I am reminded of a cartoon I saw in a book of cartoons called "Marital Blitz". The couple were in bed and the woman had a big pile of blankets while the man was trying to grab just one! In any case, some people don't sleep so well in the summer. Research indicates that a temperature between 15-19°C is best, while temperatures above 23°C or below 12°C can be disruptive to sleep.

Also we need to associate the bedroom with sleep. For example, we don't have arguments in the bedroom as it is not a good idea to go to bed angry. Nor should we work there using our bedroom as an office or using the computer late at night, as the screen creates blue light, which affects the sleep cycle. Have the computer elsewhere, or at least have the lid down. We need to use the bedroom for just sleep and intimacy. A growing problem is the intrusion of the cellphone or i-phone into sleep time. Switch it off. Most smartphones have light settings that block blue light by rendering the phone completely red or grey, which could be helpful in the evening.

As we prepare for sleep, we need to take some time to relax properly before going to bed (e.g., switch off the cell phone and computer screen). A warm bath at night (perhaps with a few drops of lavender oil in it) can be helpful to ease any stress or aches and pains. Having a fixed routine can prepare the mind for sleep. For example it is not a good idea to do anything late at night that stimulates adrenaline (e.g., watch an exciting movie or sports game on TV). Also it helps to start reducing the level of illumination early in the evening. Darkness begins to bring on the production of melatonin that tells the body to get ready for sleep. That is why the bedroom needs to be dark enough, otherwise it might be necessary to use some sort of eye covering.

Clearly quietness needs to be achieved, using ear plugs if necessary, though one can get used to certain types of noise (e.g., traffic noise). The hum of a fan can be soothing as it helps to drown out distracting noises, or it can be disturbing at first. Music may be helpful but it should switch off after about 45 minutes as it can disturb deep sleep. There are a number of tapes and CDs on the market that might be useful. If the slightest noise tends to wake you up it might be helpful to make a sleep affirmation like I will sleep deeply and easily throughout the night. Some people like to read for a short while before sleeping. Of course this involves some light stimulation and the reading matter has to be suitable.

When sleeping, it is best not to be too close to electromagnetic radiation as it can interfere with the production of melatonin. For example, having an illuminated electric clock no closer than a metre (or three feet) and not sleeping with the electric blanket on. If you are having sleep problems it might help to move the clock so you can't see it as it might make you anxious.

3.2.2 Sleeping positions

Scientists have found that most people sleep in one of six different sleeping positions, but which is the best sleeping position? The most common and best all-round position for good circulation and less strain on core body parts is the foetal position, which is sleeping on one's side with knees bent and arms out. As a variation arms can be down, though lying on an arm can cause pins and needles. A good position for back discs, muscle, and ligaments is again sleeping on one's side but now with legs straight and arms out, and trying not to bend forward too much. Some find sleeping on their back with legs and arms out in a sprawled position more comfortable, though it can lead to snoring. Some people sleep on their fronts with head turned and arms up on the pillow. This is not such a good position due to the 90 degree neck angle.

What about pillow position? If sleeping on one's side there should be a pillow under the head and neck, and between the knees to open the hips and prevent knees from pressing together (also for hip and knee replacements—I have both). For back sleeping there should be a pillow under the head and one beneath the knees to relieve pressure on the lower back. Finally, for sleeping on one's stomach, place a pillow under the head and under the hips to take stress off the lower back and neck.

3.2.3 Food and Drink

What and when we eat can also affect our body clocks. Eating at the 'wrong' time of the day (or night) can increase the risk of obesity, insulin resistance, and increased fat storage and inflammation. Snacking or grazing between meals instead of having a fasting period also dampens down the effect of our body clocks. For example, not eating after an evening meal until breakfast the next day, or not eating late at night can help with weight control. It can be helpful to have a decent fasting time period such as 12 hours between the evening meal and breakfast for weight control. Night eating syndrome is an eating disorder that involves eating more than 25% of energy intake after dinner or waking during the night to eat, and at least twice a week. It reduces both sleep time and affects the body clock.

What about food and drink before bed? Following up on alcohol discussed in section 1.9, any alcohol should be drunk at dinner time so that the liver can process it before going to bed. It takes one hour to process one standard drink so it is important not to drink too much as alcohol interferes with the sleep stages. It may help you to fall asleep (light sleep) but you will generally wake up during the night and have your deep sleep disturbed. The organisation PRIORY, a leading independent provider of behavioural care in the UK, stated that you are supposed to have between six and seven sleep cycles at night, but you typically only have one or two when you have been drinking. Also drinking before bedtime increases alpha wave patterns in the brain—a kind of cerebral activity that usually occurs when you are awake but resting (for more technical details see Colrain, Nicholas, and Baker, 2014). Insomnia and alcoholism ofter occur together, referred to as comorbidity.

L-tryptophan

As well as being careful about alcohol, it is important to avoid caffeine, nicotine, chocolate, and large amounts of food or spicy foods that may cause stomach discomfort before going to bed (see section 1.9 about caffeine). There are some foods that may help to promote sleep. For example, cheese cubes (not cheddar with tyramine) contain L-tryptophan, a natural amino acid that has been found to help with sleep. It is essential for humans and must be obtained from one's diet as the body cannot synthesize it. Also it is a major building block for making serotonin, which can be converted in the body to melatonin. In addition to cheese, foods known to be high in tryptophan include turkey, chicken, eggs, fish, peanuts, pumpkin and sesame seeds, milk, tofu and soy, and chocolate. Alcohol robs the brain of tryptophan. Some find milk drinks, cereal, nuts and seeds, bananas, dates, honey, tuna, and eggs eaten as snacks or meals beneficial for various reasons. For example, eating a snack having a complex carbohydrate and protein before bedtime can help prevent blood glucose dips during the night. If your blood sugar levels drop while sleeping, your body releases adrenaline and cortisol thus stimulating the brain and telling your body it's time to eat. In any case, hunger should be avoided as it is hard to go to sleep if you are hungry. (Although dairy products contain a minimal amount of tryptophan, it may not be enough to affect sleep.)

Some herbal drinks can be beneficial, though for some people it may be best to avoid fluids before bedtime (e.g., prostate problems with men). The elderly have to be careful here as getting out of bed at night in the dark can be hazardous. Sitting briefly on the bed before standing up can help prevent dizziness from getting up suddenly. Very small torches (say under the pillow) are available as well as night lights, and loose mats need to be avoided. Iron deficient women tend to have more problems sleeping, so a blood test for iron levels can be helpful if sleep is a problem for them.

Medications

Some medications can interfere with sleep (e.g., some antidepressants such as prozac, steroids, some drugs for treating high blood pressure, alpha blockers for enlarged prostate, nasal decongestants that contain stimulants, and thyroid hormones). For women, sleep can be affected by pregnancy (e.g., during the last trimester), menopause, and premenstrual syndrome.

In the morning everything works efficiently for healthy people. However, as the day progresses things can start to slide. For example, those with normal blood sugar control may even register within pre-diabetic sugar levels by the evening because insulin sensitivity declines. Insulin secretion is highest at lunch time and lowest during the night when food is not expected be eaten. It declines after the body releases cortisol as part of the waking up process. Healthy eating is important for well being, and recommendations include fruit and vegetables, nuts and seeds, little red meat, reduced sugar, and appropriate fats, fibre, and protein. Drinking enough liquid is important particularly with elderly people as they tend to lose their sense of thirst.

Forcing sleep

Looking at sleep from a psychological point of view, trying to force sleep can create problems. It is better to lower adrenaline arousal first. Worrying about not getting to sleep and fighting sleeplessness will make sleeping more difficult. The key is acceptance knowing that the odd night with little sleep will not hurt you. I have personally found it important to free up my mind. If something is worrying me and there is nothing I can do about it straight away, I write it down before going to bed and then tell myself to deal with it tomorrow. In particular, I don't tell myself to try and remember something I need to do tomorrow. I make a note of it and then forget it. This topic about worry is discussed later.

One may need to address a partner's sleep problems if they are disturbing you, perhaps with snoring. We discuss snoring later in the Appendix A.5 as there are a number of methods for dealing with it other than a cork!

A helpful acronym that I have used that summarises some of the above is ASLEEP, which stands for: Avoid (drugs, nicotine, alcohol, electromagnetic radiation); Sleep (and intimacy, only in the bedroom); Leave (laptop and work out of the bedroom); Empty mind (e.g., write down things to do next day); Early rising (regular times for going to bed and getting up); and Plan bedtime routine.

3.3 WAKING DURING THE NIGHT

If you wake during the night and can't get back to sleep even after using some of the above techniques, recommendations vary, for example:

(1) Don't get up unless you must. Relax and enjoy your light sleep. This may be the only viable option if the house is cold or if getting up will disturb others.

(2) Get up and repeat your night-time routine before going to bed, or do something until sleepy.

(3) Get up, go to another room and engage in relaxing activities, but remain awake. Some might prefer to use a relaxation breathing technique (see below) or have a light snack and read or listen to quiet music, but avoiding television. After a while (15-20 minutes or so) you may feel tired enough to go to bed again. Repeat this process if necessary. This seems to be the preferred option. The idea is to break the association between bed and wakefulness.

You might need to avoid the clock by removing it or covering it up. Looking at the clock can provide mixed feelings. Waking up and finding it is still very early can be very disappointing, while waking up later can bring relief as there is not so much time to go.

If insomnia persists, a person should see a doctor just in case the sleeplessness is caused by a physical problem or a medicine, either prescribed or over-the-counter (e.g., cold/allergy medications, analgesics, and diet pills). Sleeping too much can also be a problem and may indicate a sleep disorder. Some sleep disorders are discussed in the Appendix.

3.4 BREATHING AND RELAXING TECHNIQUES

There are a number of breathing techniques and they are all based on diaphragm breathing. A lot of people breathe up in their chest, expanding the chest as they breathe in. Diaphragm breathing involves breathing in through the nose to push out the stomach. You can then breathe out through your nose by pulling in your stomach (the latter stomach action is usually omitted), or breathing out can be through the mouth, whichever is preferred.

There are essentially three stages: breath in slowly, hold, breath out slowly. The time spent in each stage depends on the reason for the breathing. For example, healing breath has been described as 5-5-5 counts, while another recommendation is 6-2-8. For sleep, Dr Andrew Weill recommends 4-7-8 counts. You close your mouth and inhale quietly through your nose to a mental count of four, then hold your breath for a count of seven, and finally exhale completely through your mouth making a whoosh sound for eight seconds in one large breath. Do four times. Weill recommends practicing the technique twice a day, for six to eight weeks until you've mastered it enough to fall asleep in just 60 seconds. Personally I prefer breathing in and out through the nose and then deepening and slowing down the breathing. However we are all different.

Diaphragm breathing can be used at any time of the day to reduce stress. It can be used along with muscle relaxation. For example, in bed at night, you can tell yourself that your body is getting heavier and heavier and also focus on a peaceful scene. During the day while sitting in a chair you can tell yourself that your arms and legs are getting heavier and heavier, and relax the facial muscles. The key is to slow down the breathing (about six breaths per minute) as it affects the vagus nerve. By repeatedly stimulating the vagus nerve during those long exhalations, slow breathing may shift the nervous system towards that more restful state, resulting in positive changes like a lower heart rate and lower blood pressure. It can certainly help with insomnia (cf. Jerath, Beveridge, and Barnes, 2019)

Mental relaxation can be induced several ways. I have already mentioned imagining a peaceful scene, and an example of such a scene is a beach where we feel the sand in our toes, see life on the beach, smell the salt air, and hear the sea (if there are waves), birds, or children playing. A similar scenario could be used for a bush scene or we can imagine a waterfall with its movement and its surrounds. The idea is to engage all the physical senses in our imagination. Self hypnosis and post hypnotic suggestions have proved useful in helping people sleep. Also we must not forget that sex promotes very deep sleep, being a pleasant hypnotic!

3.5   SLEEPING PILLS

Sleeping pills can be a helpful short term support for people with occasional sleep problems such as jet lag or a stressful event such as the death of a loved one, divorce, or a medical problem. Medications used are sedatives and hypnotics, and for an example of a list see https://sleephabits.net/sleeping-pill-names. When the problem is staying asleep, one can use a hypnotic with a slower rate of elimination, while if the problem is falling asleep, a hypnotic with a rapid onset of action is preferred. If there is depression, then an antidepressant with sedative properties can be considered (e.g., amitriptyline and nortriptyline). Melatonin, which is a brain hormone that induces sleep, is available on prescription in supplement form for the treatment of insomnia. (For more information see https://emedicine.medscape.com/article/1187829-overview.)

Jacobs (1999) noted that under certain circumstances, sleeping pills may help prevent short-term insomnia from evolving into chronic insomnia. They may also help break the cycle in chronic insomnia. Some experts suggest keeping a few pills in the medicine cabinet to provide a sense of security and minimise the fear of insomnia. Lower doses are used with elderly patients. However, sleeping pills, if used at all, should only be used for short periods of time (less than 2 weeks) as they have a "hangover" effect and some side effects. They are only moderately effective, act for a limited length of time in the night, can be addictive with a build up of tolerance, can produce withdrawal symptoms on stopping, but do not solve the sleep problem. So-called "rebound insomnia" can happen when coming off the tablets, and can also happen when taking a tablet one night leads to wakefulness the next night.

The sleep one experiences while on sleeping pills tends to be very superficial, light stage sleep. Also the sleep cycle is disrupted, so that the benefits of deep sleep and REM sleep are missing. Sleeping pills can be a short term crutch and do not solve sleep problems. If a person has been on such tablets for four or more weeks, it is important not to suddenly stop taking them. They need to talk to their doctor about how to reduce the dose slowly to avoid potentially dangerous withdrawal symptoms.

There can be some serious side effects of sleeping tablets such as dizziness, chest pains, decreased sex drive, sleepwalking, hallucinations, violent outbursts, sleep-eating, and driving while asleep. A large study in the British Medical Journal (2012) found that people who persistently take sleeping pills were four times more likely to die than those not taking sleeping pills. In fact even those who took fewer than 18 pills per year were found to have an elevated mortality risk. Furthermore, patients who took more than two sleeping pills a week over the course of a year had a 35 percent increased risk of cancer. The pills don't increase sleep time.

Sleeping pills can be a particular problem for older people as they take a longer time to break down and therefore stay in the system longer with older bodies. That makes it more likely that a user will wake up feeling confused, groggy or unsteady on the feet—exactly the kinds of problems that many older people already face even without sleeping pills. Also older people tend to be taking other medications as well (e.g., pain medication), so that interactions with other drugs can be a problem. For people over sixty the side effects of sleeping pills outweigh their small benefit and CBT-I, discussed below (section 3.8), should be used instead of pills.

Jacobs (1999) said that sleeping pills are

> no longer considered a safe or appropriate treatment for chronic insomnia
> because they can have serious side effects that far outweigh their benefits;
> ... (they) strengthen the belief that the cure for insomnia comes from
> external factors; and can lead to physical or psychological dependency,
> which can cause feelings of helplessness, loss of control, and lowered self-
> esteem.

Part of the problem is the successful marketing of the pills. Information on the downside of using sleeping tablets is available on the internet. (See http://www.darksideofsleepingpills.com by Daniel Kripke). As noted previously, the side effects can be greater for older people, and the usefulness of sleeping tablets for them is uncertain as their long term effects and interactions with other drugs are unknown.

Walker (2018) said that sleeping tablets can stop the brain cells from firing, like alcohol. If you compare natural sleeping brainwave activity with that under the newer sedatives, the largest, deepest brainwaves are missing. They can make a person groggy, forgetful and more prone to mistakes the next day. He said that some studies suggest sleeping pills may actually weaken memory connections normally made during sleep. Even worse, sleeping pills are associated with a significantly higher death rate as well as cancer (Kripke, Langer, and Kline, 2012).

3.5.1   Strategies with Sleeping Pills

Sedative-hypnotics are the most commonly prescribed drugs for insomnia. Though not usually curative, they can provide symptomatic relief when used alone or with other medication. If a person is taking them, then the following cautionary strategies are recommended:

(1) Use the smallest possible dose, and maintain at the lowest effective dose.

(2) Never use with alcohol.

(3) Use intermittently, only after two consecutive bad nights of sleep and never on consecutive nights (i.e., no more than twice a week).

(4) Avoid using for more than 2-4 weeks if possible.

(5) Don't escalate the dose and try to use sleep medications with a short half-life (hours rather than days), that is they stay in the body for only a short period of time.

(6) Allow for at least 8 hours of sleep.

(7) Avoid using in pregnant patients.

(8) Avoid using benzodiazepines if there is known or possible sleep apnea.

(9) When the problem is falling asleep, consider hypnotics with a rapid onset of action, while if the problem is staying asleep, consider a hypnotic with a slower rate of elimination.

(10) If there is depression, an antidepressant with sedative properties can be used.

If a client is wanting to cut out a regular use of sleeping tablets, Jacobs suggests the following strategies:

(1) Start the reduction program when life is not too busy or stressful.

(2) Begin by cutting the dose in half on one of the medication nights. Choose a low stress night such as a weekend night.

(3) Once sleeping reasonably well on this dosage, try a reduction on another low stress night suitably spaced from the first. Continue until all nights are on half dosage.

(4) Repeat the process by steadily cutting out all doses.

(5) Don't rush the process as it may take a while, especially with long term use.

There are some safe, natural alternatives to sleeping pills. Below are five natural sleep aids that you can get without a prescription. No doubt there are others on the market, and care is needed if using them.

3.5.2 Natural Alternatives

Melatonin: You may have heard about this one but not perhaps realised how helpful it can be as a supplement, especially with the elderly. The pineal gland produces melatonin in the absence of light. As already discussed, it regulates your natural sleep cycle, which helps you fall asleep and stay asleep. The most important thing to understand about melatonin is that it is a hormone. So one needs to be careful when supplementing with it. Too much can do more harm than good. Its usefulness is uncertain and its long term effects and interactions with other drugs is unknown. It does have few side effects but is not addictive, and simply helps an individual fall asleep more quickly, rather than tossing and turning after they go to bed. It does not improve the quality of sleep once a person falls asleep so that the supplement is only a temporary remedy to be used in moderation. Taking too much may lead the body to stop producing melatonin naturally as it comes to rely on the supplement. Instead of artificial sources, melatonin is found naturally in foods like walnuts, ginger, asparagus, bananas, and tart cherries described below. A few almonds and walnuts (both containing tryptophan) in the evening can be helpful. Kiwi fruit also contains tryptophan, and along with a number of other good substances such as its high folate and potassium levels can be good to have some time before bedtime.

Tart Cherry Juice: This is an excellent, natural source of melatonin. Tart cherries contain more melatonin than any other food. They are loaded with antioxidants and fibre, so they make a great snack or juice no matter how many "zzz's" you are catching each night.

L-Tryptophan: L-Tryptophan, which we have already mentioned is an amino acid that is essential, meaning the body cannot create it itself so that it must be obtained from the foods we eat.

Valerian: Valerian root is a herb that grows in Europe and Asia. It may not smell great, but people have been using it since the 2nd century to help them sleep, which says a lot about its effect. Recent studies demonstrate the effectiveness of valerian as a sleep aid. One study shows that valerian root extract taken twice a day helps postmenopausal women have a more restful sleep. However it does have side effects with some people, and a medical practitioner should be consulted before using it.

5-HTP: Its full name 5-Hydroxytryptophancan be a real mouthful, but the idea behind its use is simple. 5-HTP is a chemical that the body can make after having L-Tryptophan. It converts to serotonin, which may help one to fall asleep faster. Taking 5-HTP as a supplement is also known to fight depression and the effects of fibromyalgia.

Lemon balm: Lemon balm (*Melissa officinalis*) is a lemon-scented herb that comes from the same family as mint. The herb is native to Europe, North Africa, and West Asia, but it is grown around the world. It has a number of physical benefits and can be combined with valerian to help with sleep problems.

There are some nutrients that may be helpful for sleep such as calcium (e.g., leafy greens and sesame seeds) and magnesium (e.g., leafy greens, seafood, legumes, nuts, and seeds), both of which promote muscle relaxation and nerve sedating. Then there is vitamin C (e.g., oranges, broccoli etc.), Omega 3 fatty acids (e.g., fish, the precursor ALA from flaxseed, leafy greens, cruciferous vegetables, and beans), iron (e.g., greens, beans, and dark chocolate), potassium (e.g., sweet potatoes, watermelon, beets, and many others), vitamin D3 (sunshine!), and vitamin B12 (e.g., organ meats, eggs, and fatty fish). There are many other sources, and if sleep is a problem this topic of diet is worth looking into with regard to natural nutrients.

Lack of sleep can cause depression, and depression an affect sleep. We now take a close look at the effect of depression.

3.6   DEPRESSION AND SLEEP

A change in one's normal sleep pattern, with either sleeping too much (approximately 15% of sleep problems) or too little, and having broken sleep throughout the night, can be a very useful diagnostic aid for depression. Many depressed people complain that their minds go round and round when they try to go off to sleep. A person suffering from depression has the pattern reversed with regard to REM and non REM sleep: REM sleep happens much more quickly after first falling asleep and decreases towards the morning. Depressed people have excessive REM sleep, and antidepressants suppress REM sleep, delay its onset, and decrease its duration thus helping to normalise the sleep pattern.

Excessive dreaming

What about excessive dreaming? Dreaming seems to be a kind of "clearing-house" for our brains, and it can be argued that depressed people do so much worrying and negative thinking during the day that there is an overload of dreaming that uses a lot of energy in the brain. There is then less of the recuperative deeper sleep so that they wake up exhausted and unable to get going. According to this view, people generate their own depression and the key to overcoming this problem is to change daytime thinking and ruminating. Non-sedating antidepressants used in the daytime will often resolve the sleep problem, though some can cause sleeplessness. Some antidepressant medications that have a sedating effect (e.g. amitriptyline and nortriptyline) can be also used in the evening.

3.7   JET LAG

Jet lag can certainly play havoc with sleep. If you are going to spend several days in a different time zone, you need to start adjusting meals and bedtime to the new time zone before leaving home, then adjust meal times and sleep schedule to the new time zone immediately on arrival. If the adjustment is several hours earlier, we can use sunlight and activity or a short nap to stay awake for the longer day. We note that our natural circadian rhythm is, in fact, slightly longer than 24 hours (24.5). I always found it difficult to adjust to the reverse situation of a shortened day as there is a tendency to go to bed very late in the new time zone, but getting up at the usual time. At night it is still early in the old time zone so it is hard to get the body temperature down at bedtime in the new time zone. Also, when flying, the stomach expands slightly, which affects eating schedules. The key is to adjust the body temperature cycle as soon as possible. It is a lot worse if you are away for only a short time so you have to adjust back again. According to Walker (2018:25) it takes a day's adjustment for ever hour difference in time zone.

3.8   COGNITIVE BEHAVIOURAL THERAPY FOR INSOMNIA (CBT-I)

Internationally, sleeping pills are not the No. 1 treatment. Numerous clinical studies have proven CBT for insomnia (CBT-I) is superior to sleeping pills for onset, length, and quality of sleep. Some sleep clinics provide CBT-I in New Zealand. In Australia, GPs have the option of referring a patient with insomnia to a registered psychologist for treatment under the Medicare mental health care programme. In the UK, the National Health Service covers CBT-I with or without a GP referral. In CBT-I the patient works with a therapist over a number of weeks, building on basic principles such as reducing screen time, caffeine and alcohol, regular bedtime and wake-up, going to bed only when sleepy and not remaining in bed if awake with methods individualised for the patient, their problems, and lifestyle. All of which is part of what is called sleep hygiene discussed above and in Appendix A1.

One of the main goals of CBT-I is to reduce the amount of time that people spend awake in bed. That means not using the bed for reading and particularly work, and perhaps getting out of bed if it feels like sleep isn't coming. If they can spend less time struggling for sleep, even hard-core insomniacs can feel more confident when they get under the covers. One aspect of this is the technique of sleep deprivation. Here the idea is to get up the same time every morning, but go to bed late enough so that most of bedtime is sleeping, i.e., high sleep efficiency (see section 2.2). Another technique called paradoxical intention is where you try to stay awake as long as possible.

An essential part of CBT-I is to change our beliefs about sleep. For example, we need to avoid faulty thinking and negative thoughts about sleep. We can counter "I need at least eight hours of sleep tonight to cope the next day" with "I don't necessarily need eight hours as everybody is different" or with "I will naturally catch up on my sleep over the next few nights." Another thought might be: "I didn't sleep a wink last night." However, insomniacs are generally not accurate in estimating how much sleep they actually get as they tend to over-estimate how long they are awake during the night. A common thought is: "How will I function today after such a horrible night of sleep?" This can be countered with the fact that provided I get "core" sleep (deep sleep), which is about five and a half hours, I will be able to function adequately the next day. Get the idea?

If you're lying awake with brain whirring, then rather than attempting any particular exercise or counting sheep (which Oxford University has officially debunked for its sleep-inducing abilities) is to stop actively trying to sleep, as this will only make matters worse. We need to avoid getting into that mindset of counting how many hours we have got left before we need to be up and worrying about how we will feel tomorrow. Instead we can try thinking about a time we had little or no sleep, but managed to perform satisfactorily the next day. The fact we have coped before means we can cope again. Having shown resilience before means we can show it again. With this in mind we are much more likely to calm our brain and let sleep enter. The key is acceptance knowing that the odd night with little sleep will not kill us.

In addition to working through CBT-I with a therapist there may be other psychological aspects that need to be dealt with such as what led to the insomnia in the first place. For example there may be a need to reduce stress, anger, and negative self-talk, and enjoy humour. Psychological stress is a major cause of insomnia as the sympathetic nervous system becomes overactive raising blood pressure, the heart rate, the metabolic rate, and internal temperature including the brain. As already noted previously, for sleep to happen the core body temperature needs to drop by a few degrees Fahrenheit or a degree Centigrade. Stress also raises the levels of stress hormones such as cortisol and associated brain transmitters, which will keep you awake.

Having discussed a range of strategies I have now put them all together along with further suggestions in the Appendix A1 for easy reference. Also there I discuss some of the major sleep disorders.

SLEEP TIPS AND DISORDERS

A.1   SLEEP PROGRAMME

A number of guides to a good night's sleep (sleep hygiene) are available and the following are drawn from a number of sources, not necessarily in a time order. The list also provides a summary of chapter 3, and one can select what is appropriate.

- Have a good supporting mattress and pillow.

- Avoid being too close to electromagnetic radiation as it can interfere with the production of melatonin. For example, have an illuminated electric clock no closer than a metre (three feet) and do not sleep with an electric blanket on.

- Develop regular sleep habits. This means waking up at the same time every morning, even on weekends. Avoid snoozing then as it can make you more tired. Also avoid staying in bed in the morning to catch up on sleep. The aim is to sleep enough to feel refreshed the following day, but not spending more time in bed than needed. Aim for about 8 hours, or at least 7-9 hours.

- Keep a regular daytime schedule. Regular times for meals, medications, chores, and other activities helps keep the inner body clock running smoothly.

- An outdoor morning run or walk can lower blood pressure, and some sunlight will help with the diurnal cycle. You may be able to walk to work, or at least get off public transport some stops earlier, and use stairs rather than lifts at work. Also stand up when on the phone and don't sit for too long a period (less than an hour) without movement. Some use a fitness tracker to stay active during the day and recommend so many steps a day, while others go to a gym. A lunchtime walk may be possible, or else exercise in the late afternoon or early evening (but not later than 6-7 pm, or four to six hours before bedtime). However, whatever the method, having a fitness programme is essential.

- Have a nutritious breakfast.

- Periodically rest your eyes if you are glued to a computer screen at work (and perhaps do some shoulder exercises).

- Get outside for lunch for some light exposure if possible. In any case have a relaxed lunch to lower stress levels. Exposure to bright sunlight during the day can help with sleep.

- Generally avoid daytime naps. However, a short nap during the day can be helpful as there is a dip in body temperature after lunch. If you must sleep during the day keep it short. It is best to restrict it to less than 30 minutes early in the day to avoid going into a deep sleep cycle. However, with severe fatigue a longer sleep might be needed. Avoid napping after 3 pm.

- Avoid caffeine after lunch or at least late afternoon, remembering that it has a 6 hour half-life. Caffeine acts as a diuretic in the body by pulling water from cells and tissues leading to more urinating at night.

- Switch off from work when it is time to go home so you don't take work home with you (this is not always possible, but you have to switch off sometime). It is no good venting your frustration from work by kicking the cat or yelling at family members.

- Eat your last meal at least three hours before going to bed. However, do not go to bed hungry, but do not eat a big meal near bedtime either. Also avoid caffeine, nicotine, chocolates, and large amounts of food or spicy foods that may cause stomach discomfort before going to bed. Avoid alcohol as it interferes with sleep patterns. Medscape, the online medical information source, recommends avoiding alcohol within 6 hours of bedtime. Remember that one standard drink takes one hour to metabolise.

- Start to limit fluids to prevent interrupted sleep, especially men with a prostate problem.

- Turn off all backlit screens (mobile, laptop, TV etc.) 90 minutes before getting into bed. Cellphones are blamed for poor sleep. For example, young people are often felt pressured to reply to texts immediately, regardless of the time of day or night. There is a tendency for many of them to sleep with phones nearby and therefore get woken up by alerts from incoming texts.

- Having a warm shower can help as your body cools down quickly afterwards bringing on sleep. A warm bath (perhaps with a few drops of lavender oil in it) can be helpful to ease stress.

- Avoid stimulating activities prior to bedtime (e.g., vigorous exercise, watching exciting TV, discussing or reviewing finances, or discussing stressful issues with a spouse or partner, or ruminating about them yourself).

- Free up your mind. If something is worrying you and there is nothing you can do about it straight away, try writing it down before going to bed. Jot down all worries or things that need doing the next day to get them out of your head before going to bed, and then tell yourself to deal with them tomorrow.

- Slow down and unwind before bed beginning at least 30 minutes before bedtime (a light snack may be helpful); create a bedtime ritual such as getting ready for bed, wearing night clothes, listening to relaxing music, or reading a magazine, newspaper, or book.

- Keep the bedroom dark, quiet, (or else use a mask and ear plugs if not possible), and at a comfortable temperature. If the bedroom temperature is too hot it will raise body temperature and affect the sleep cycle. One can get used to a certain types of noise (e.g., traffic noise). The hum of a fan can be soothing as it helps to drown out distracting noises. Music may be helpful but it should switch off after about 45 minutes as it can disturb deep sleep. If the slightest noise wakes you up it might be helpful to make a sleep affirmation like "I will sleep deeply and easily throughout the night."

- Do not use your bedroom as an office (e.g., have the computer elsewhere). Use the bedroom only for sleep and intimacy. This will strengthen the association of the bed with sleep.

- Do not read (though some people find this helpful), write, eat, watch TV, talk on the phone, or play cards in bed. This is referred to as stimulus control.

- Avoid sleeping on the sofa and then going to bed later in the night.

- Reduce the level of illumination early in the evening; again stimulus control. Darkness begins the production of melatonin that tells the body to get ready for sleep.

- Learn a relaxation technique, e.g., diaphragm breathing, relaxing tense muscles, and picturing a peaceful scene to distract a racing or obsessed mind. Such techniques can produce a brain-wave pattern similar to stage 1 sleep. There are also a number of tapes and CDs on the market that might be useful. Some find meditation helpful.

- Do not force yourself to sleep; if you are unable to fall asleep within 15-30 minutes, get up and do something relaxing until sleepy (e.g., read a book in a dimly lit room, watch a non-stimulating TV program); avoid watching the clock or worrying about the perceived consequences of not getting enough sleep.

- You may have to address your partner's sleep problems such as snoring if they are disturbing you.

- Remember that some medications can interfere with sleep.

- If insomnia is a problem, then a sleep diary can be a good idea for keeping track of one's sleep patterns. Information recorded could include bed hours, amount of sleep, time to get off to sleep, breaks in sleep, quality of sleep, feelings, negative sleep thoughts, what they did when awake during the night, what they did and what food and drink they consumed before going to bed, and medications used. This sounds a lot of information. However, the aim is not to get hung up with recording during the night as clock watching can be counter productive, but simply to get a rough idea of sleep patterns.

Much of the above has already been discussed in greater detail in chapter 3 and elsewhere, and one hat does not to fit all heads. However most people find it helpful to have a list. Clearly people will modify the above such as some of the times to suit their own circumstances and lifestyle. The idea of producing such a list is to emphasise the need for a structured programme and having a list to work from. Further information is available from the American Academy of Sleep Medicine Sleep Education site, for example.

A helpful acronym that summarises some of the above is ASLEEP, which stands for: **A**void (drugs, nicotine, alcohol, electromagnetic radiation); **S**leep (and intimacy) only in the bedroom; **L**eave (laptop and work out of the bedroom); **E**mpty mind (e.g., write down things to do next day); **E**arly rising (same time every day); and **P**lan bedtime routine.

A.2 SLEEP DISORDERS

As there are over 60 known sleep disorders currently defined by the American Academy of Sleep Medicine we look at just the more well-known ones. The term used is *primary* sleep disorders, which include only those not attributable to another medical or psychiatric condition. There are two main categories, insomnia and excessive daytime sleepiness, and include insomnia disorder, hypersomnolence disorder, narcolepsy, obstructive sleep apnea hypopnea syndrome, central sleep apnea syndrome, and the parasomnias. They are commonly encountered and can be comorbid (coexisting) with many psychiatric disorders.

If your GP thinks that you could have a sleep disorder, you might be referred to a sleep specialist or sleep clinic for further assessment. A polysomnography, which is a comprehensive diagnostic test conducted in sleep clinics (cf. section 1.13), may be used if sleep apnoea, discussed below, is suspected as the cause of insomnia. For insomnia to be considered a disorder, it should be accompanied by daytime tiredness, loss of concentration, irritability, worries about sleep, loss of motivation, or other evidence of daytime impairment that is associated with the sleep difficulty. We have already mentioned some of the signposts for insomnia in chapter 1. However we now take a more clinical approach in what follows.

A.3   INSOMNIA

According to the *Diagnostic and Statistical Manual of Mental Disorders, Fifth Edition (DSM-5)*, insomnia is dissatisfaction with sleep quantity associated with one (or more) of the following symptoms (and independent of any coexisting conditions, being a condition in its own right):

- Difficulty initiating sleep.

- Difficulty maintaining sleep, characterised by frequent awakenings or problems returning to sleep after awakenings.

- Early-morning awakening with inability to return to sleep.

These generally agree with the *International Classification of Sleep Disorders, Third Edition (ICSD-3)*. Further criteria that need to be satisfied are:

- The sleep disturbance causes clinically significant distress or impairments in social, occupational, educational, academic, behavioural, or other important areas of functioning.

- The sleep difficulty occurs at least 3 nights per week.

- The sleep difficulty is present for at least 3 months.

- The sleep difficulty occurs despite adequate opportunity for sleep

- The insomnia cannot be explained by, and does not occur exclusively during the course of, another sleep-wake disorder.

- The insomnia is not attributable to the physiological effects of a drug abuse or medication.

- Coexisting mental disorders and medical conditions do not adequately explain the predominant complaint of insomnia.

Doctor Jasvinder Chawla, writing for Medscape (Sept. 11, 2018), who listed the above, described a program from the American Academy of Sleep Medicine (AASM) for carrying a diagnosis of insomnia (https://emedicine.medscape.com/article/1187829-overview), which is included in the list below. The guideline consensus is that, at a minimum, patients with insomnia (or excessive daytime sleepiness) should begin with the following evaluations:

(1) Obtain a sleep history covering the timing of insomnia, the patient's sleep habits (commonly referred to as sleep hygiene

discussed in section A.1), the presence or absence of symptoms of sleep disorders associated with insomnia, and a thorough medical history. The role and timing of any naps can also provide helpful information.

(2) Obtain a psychological history to screen for any psychiatric disorders (especially heritable or family conditions), looking particularly for any anxiety and depression. A general medical and psychiatric questionnaire can detect comorbid (other additional) disorders.

(3) Obtain a complete physical examination looking for underlying medical disorders predisposing to insomnia. For example, appropriate serum laboratory tests can be made such as a blood test to check for thyroid problems.

(4) A social history can also be obtained by considering any recent stresses leading to short term insomnia, past stresses, medical illnesses causing chronic insomnia, and uses of tobacco, caffeinated products, alcohol, and illegal drugs.

(5) A medication history is also important as some medications commonly cause insomnia such as beta blockers (e.g., for high blood pressure), clonidine, theophylline, certain antidepressants (e.g., protriptyline and fluoxetine, also called prozac), decongestants, stimulants, and some over-the-counter and herbal remedies. However, there are also sedating antidepressants that can be used in the treatment of insomnia.

(6) It is helpful to include a 2-week sleep log or diary to define sleep-wake patterns and their variability.

(7) A sleepiness assessment, such as the Epworth Sleepiness Scale (section A.7 below) can be used.

(8) It can be helpful to have a bed partner interview if appropriate, as self assessment is not always easy or reliable.

Before moving on to other sleep disorders, mention should be made of another insomnia problem. There are basically three types of insomnia problems, namely, having difficulty falling asleep, failing to stay asleep with waking during the night, or waking too early in the morning. There is a fourth rare problem called paradoxical insomnia where a person's brain stays alert while their body sleeps so that they are in a state between sleep and wakefulness. Those with this problem often report spending hours lying awake at night, even though, to others, they appear to be sleeping. They overestimate the time it takes for them to fall asleep and underestimate their total sleep time.

A.4 PRIMARY SLEEP DISORDERS CAUSING INSOMNIA

As already noted, primary sleep disorders include those not attributable to another medical or psychiatric condition (Khoury and Doghramji (2015). In this section we first consider three important sleep disorders: restless legs syndrome, obstructive sleep apnea/hypopnea syndrome, and circadian rhythm disorders. These are discussed below and such sleep disorders are part of what are known as parasomnias.

A.4.1   Restless Legs Syndrome (RLS)

RLS is defined as an urge to move one's legs, usually accompanied by uncomfortable and unpleasant physical sensations in the legs. Many people have experienced this at some stage in their life, and it can be very disturbing when it occurs. You feel like taking off your legs and putting them on the mantel piece, or some such place. The symptoms begin or worsen during periods of rest or inactivity such as lying or sitting, and are partially or totally relieved by moving, massaging or stretching limbs, at least as long as the restlessness continues. In the past I found knee bending with partial squats helpful. Symptoms are worse or occur only in the evening or at night. It can be associated with periodic limb movement disorder, which is characterised by repetitive periodic leg movements that occur during sleep.

Up to 19% of pregnant women develop RLS during pregnancy and generally women are affected more than twice as often as men. It important to move around during the day, e.g., stand up to improve circulation and use leg stretches regularly during the day, run on the spot for a few minutes, have a walk at lunch time, use a leg massage, perhaps use ice packs, and if it happens in bed, lightly massage the legs or get up and move around. Low iron levels may be responsible. The key is movement, and of course relaxation techniques will help.

A.4.2   Obstructive Sleep Apnea (OSA)

This comparatively common sleep disorder causes one's breathing to stop briefly while sleeping due to the upper airways getting blocked. The pauses in breathing wake a person up from deep sleep, and this happens several times during an hour. The majority of those suffering from this condition do not remember these troublesome interruptions, but they do feel tired during the day, besides being depressed and irritated, and possibly underproductive. Summing up, the symptoms include:

- Regular pauses in breathing during sleep.

- Snorting, choking or gasping during sleep.

- Tiredness during waking hours regardless of how long one has slept.

- Awakening with chest pains, nasal congestion, dry throat, or shortness of breath.

If your child snores, ask your paediatrician about it as children can also have OSA. Nose and throat problems, such as enlarged tonsils and obesity, often can narrow a child's airway, which can lead to your child developing OSA.

Sleep apnea can be a serious and sometimes fatal sleep disorder, but it does not mean that you will choke to death. If you think that you or someone close to you is suffering from this condition, go and see a doctor immediately. Yale University sleep expert Dr. Meir Kryger writes in "The Mystery of Sleep" that moderate alcohol consumption before bed can also exacerbate the effects of sleep apnea, where the airways are temporarily blocked while you sleep. That is backed up by a study in 2018 that reviewed 21 experiments over 30 years, between 1985 and 2015, and found that obstructive sleep apnea was more likely in people who drank moderate or heavy amounts of alcohol.

Being overweight or obese is a major risk factor in suffering from obstructive sleep apnoea so that the first thing to try is weight loss, as that often improves sleep. Also there is Continuous Positive Airway Pressure (CPAP), which uses a mask-like device to deliver a small increase in airway pressure to stop snoring and sleep apnoea.

A.4.3 Narcolepsy

This is a sleep disorder which causes uncontrollable and excessive daytime drowsiness and emerges between the age of ten and twenty years. There is a genetic basis, which can be tested for (e.g., HLA2 and HLADQ B1*60) that could be due to a mutation as it is not inherited, but there are other unknown factors. Narcolepsy is a result of a dysfunctional brain mechanism, specifically the mechanism responsible for controlling waking and sleeping. What happens is that the body attacks the immune system and depletes the hypocretins, which are neurotransmitters in the brain that help sustain alertness and prevent REM sleep from occurring at the wrong times. If a person suffers from narcolepsy, they might suffer from "sleep attacks" mid-speech, mid-work, and even mid-driving! It is a dangerous. Unfortunately there is no cure at present, but there are some medications that can at least help. Common symptoms are:

- Hallucinating when feeling sleepy or dreaming before fully asleep.

- Sudden feelings of weakness/losing muscle controls when one is angry, laughing or otherwise emotionally affected.

- Dreaming as soon as one drifts off, or experiencing strong dreams.

- Feelings of paralysis/lost movement when one is either waking up or going to sleep.

Walker (2018:247) explains it in three core symptoms: (1) excessive daytime sleepiness, the first symptom to appear, (2) sleep paralysis, when waking up from sleep, and (3) cataplexy, when there is a sudden loss of muscle control ranging

> from slight weakness wherein the head droops, the face sags, the jaw drops, and speech becomes slurred to a buckling of the knees or a sudden and immediate loss of all muscle tone, resulting in total collapse on the spot.

Remember that in REM sleep the brain paralises the body to stop one acting out their dreams. However, the paralysis can linger on when awake on very rare occasions even with a person without narcolepsy. With narcolepsy it occurs much more frequently and severely.

A.4.4 Circadian Rhythm Disorders

These disorders include the following:

Advanced sleep phase syndrome: Here patients feel sleepy earlier than their desired bedtime (e.g., 8 p.m.) and they wake up earlier than they would like (e.g., 4-5 a.m.). This condition is more common in the elderly.

Delayed sleep phase syndrome: In delayed sleep phase syndrome, patients do not feel sleepy until much later than the desired bedtime, and they wake up later than desired or socially acceptable. The condition often begins in adolescence (though many outgrow it) and may be associated with a family history in up to 40% of patients. These patients report difficulty falling asleep at usually socially desired bedtimes and complain of excessive daytime sleepiness during school or work. When it is possible for them to follow their own hours, they will get into a proper sleep schedule.

Shift-work sleep disorder: This is excessive sleepiness that typically is temporally related to a recurring work schedule that overlaps with the usual sleep time. It can happen with an early shift e.g., starting at 4-6 a.m. where patients are anxious about waking up in time for their early shift, particularly when they have a rotating-shift schedule. Alternatively it can happen with evening shifts that end at 11 p.m. when the person may need some time to wind down from work before retiring to bed.

Irregular sleep-wake rhythm: This can occur with people who have poor sleep habits, particularly those who live or work alone with minimal exposure to light, activity, and social cues.

A.5   SNORING

Nearly everyone snores now and then (e.g., nasal congestion), but for some people it can be a chronic problem, and a disaster for a couple sharing the same bed. Snoring can be caused by a number of factors such as the anatomy of one's mouth and sinuses, alcohol consumption (which relaxes the throat muscles and decreases one's natural defences against airway obstruction), allergies (perhaps one might need to change their pillow because of, say, dust mites), a cold, and one's weight. Some people have a low, thick soft palate that can narrow their airway, while the uvula (the triangular piece of tissue hanging from the soft palate) can be elongated causing an obstruction. People who are overweight may have extra tissues in the back of their throats that may narrow their airways. Sleep deprivation can lead to further throat relaxation, while sleeping on one's back allows gravity to affect the throat and narrow the airway

According to the Sleep Health Foundation, snoring is a common condition that affects 40% of adult men and 30% of adult women. It signals that something may be wrong with the way one is breathing as they sleep. When a person goes to sleep and progresses from light sleep to deep sleep, the muscles in the body relax, including the muscles that hold the airway open when awake. In some people, the airway is narrow enough so that the normal suction of breathing in causes the airway to vibrate. Nerves can then send a signal to the brain that the snoring is actually the beginning of choking. This causes the brain to go on alert, and the coming out of deep sleep into light sleep, which allows the airway to pop back open again. So the airway always opens up, but at the cost of disrupted deep sleep.

Some people snore so badly that the airway is sucked shut over and over throughout the night, even a 100 times. This is Obstructive Sleep Apnoea mentioned above. Because sleep apnoea is relatively common you cannot tell easily if someone is just snoring or if they have sleep apnoea. Weight gain can make the snoring more problematic.

A Massey University study in New Zealand found that one in five New Zealand women are loud snorers in the final months of pregnancy, and they have an increased risk of depression. As already mentioned above, alcohol can cause the same muscle relaxation.

Summing up then is a list of possible lifestyle changes to reduce snoring.

Lose weight. People who are overweight are two times more likely to snore than those who are not. The reason is simple as overweight people carry extra fat around their necks which narrows their airways and causes them to snore.

Cut down on alcohol and cigarettes. Alcohol relaxes your throat muscles while regular smokers are likely to snore. Smoking irritates the throat tissues leading to inflammation, and hence to snoring.

Sleep on your side. Sleeping on your back can cause your airway to become blocked or narrowed. Old habits die hard so the odds are that as you drift deeper into sleep you would roll onto your back again. A body pillow can help with this or sowing tennis balls on the back of your pyjamas!

Elevate your head while you sleep. If sleeping on your side does not work you might need to prop up your head a little bit to ease breathing and open up the airways.

Stay well hydrated. This helps as secretions in the nose and soft palate become stickier when one is dehydrated, which increases the possibility of snoring.

A humidifier in the bedroom. This can be helpful as the added moisture in the air will help lubricate your throat.

Exercise your tongue and throat muscles. They may be too relaxed. Singing is good for throat exercise. A tongue exercise is to place the tip of your tongue behind the top of your teeth and slide it back and forth for a couple of minutes a day.

Examine your diet. Cut down on inflammatory food. This effect will vary from person to person. For example some people might need to avoid gluten or some dairy products. There is a hydrogen test that can help determine if you have an allergy.

Inhaling steam before bedtime. This can open the airways.

Methods for helping with snoring include surgery (which may not help), using a mouth guard-like device that suits some people called a mandibular splint that pulls the bottom jaw forward during sleep thus opening the airway to help prevent the tongue from collapsing into the throat. This reduces the risk of soft tissues falling close enough together to vibrate. As noted above, another technique is to use Continuous Positive Airway Pressure (CPAP), which uses a mask-like device to deliver a small increase in airway pressure to stop snoring and sleep apnoea. Although there are several other gadgets available, and the internet provides many examples, care is needed as many stop-snoring aids are marketed without scientific studies to support their claims. Although medical devices and surgery are available that may reduce disruptive snoring, they are not suitable or necessary for everyone who snores.

A.6   SOMNAMBULISM

This term refers to sleep (*somnus*) disorders that involve some movement (*ambulation*). Most episodes of this condition are harmless and not pathological, and involve doing physical things in your sleep such as sleepwalking and sleep talking. They are common in the adult population and even more common with children as they have more deep NREM sleep. These activities actually occur during the deepest stage of non-dreaming (NREM) sleep, and not during dream (REM) sleep, when perhaps a spike of brain activity induces a state of being between asleep and awake. In spite of the physical movement, the brain is sound asleep with slow electrical waves of deep NREM sleep. Walker (2018:240) notes that most somnambulism episodes are considered benign and do not require intervention.

A.7   EPWORTH SLEEPINESS SCALE

The following is a useful questionnaire about sleep. Scoring is done as follows: 0=Would **never** doze/fall asleep;1=**Slight** chance of dozing/falling asleep; 2=**Moderate** chance of dozing/falling asleep; and 3=**Strong** chance of dozing/falling asleep, for the following situations:

- Sitting and reading

- Watching the television
- Sitting, inactive in a public place (eg., a theatre or meeting)
- As a passenger in a car for an hour without a break
- Lying down to rest in the afternoon when circumstances permit
- Sitting and talking to someone
- Sitting quietly after a lunch without alcohol
- In a car, while stopping for a few minutes in traffic

Perhaps I should add "reading this book" to the list! A total score greater than 10 is considered abnormal, while a total score greater than 16 indicates pathological daytime sleepiness. In conclusion, if you have a sleep problem you need a plan. It is hoped that this book will help provide one.

Ancoli-Israel, S., Cole, R., Alessi, C., Chambers, M., Moorcroft, W., and Pollak, C. P. (2003). The role of actigraphy in the study of sleep and circadian rhythms. American Academy of Sleep Medicine Review Paper. *SLEEP*, **26** (3), 342–392.

Cappuccio, F. P., D'Elia, L., Strazzullo, P., and Miller, M. A. (2010). Sleep duration and all-cause mortality: A systematic review and meta-analysis of prospective studies. *SLEEP*, **33** (5), 585–592.

Chawla, J. (2018). Insomnia. *Medscape*, Sept. 11

Colrain, I. M., Nicholas, C. L., and Baker, F. C. (2014). Alcohol and the sleeping brain. *Handbook of Clinical Neurology*, **125**, 415–431.

Ford, E. S., Cunningham, T. J, and Croft, J. B. (2015). Trends in self-reported sleep duration among US adults from 1985 to 2012. *SLEEP*, **38** (5), 829–832.

Gallicchio, L. and Kalesan B. (2009). Sleep duration and mortality: a systematic review and meta-analysis. *Journal of Sleep Research*, **18**, 148–158.

Gander, P., O' Keefe., K., et al. (2019). Fatigue and nurses' work patterns: An online questionnaire survey. *International Journal of Nursing Studies*, **98**, 67–74.

Hirshkowitz, M., Whiton, K., et al. (2015). National Sleep Foundation's sleep time duration recommendations: methodology and results summary. *Sleep Health*, **1** (1), 40–43.

Hublin, C., Partinen, M., Koskenvuo, M., and Kaprio, J. (2007). Sleep and mortality: a population-based 22-year follow-up study. *SLEEP*, **30** (10), 1245–1253.

Jerath, R., Beveridge, C., and Barnes, V. A. (2019). Self-regulation of breathing as an adjunctive treatment of insomnia. *Frontiers in Psychiatry*, https://doi.org/10.3389/fpsyt.2018.00780.

Jacobs, G. D. (1999). *Say Goodnight to Insomnia: The Six Week, Drug-Free Program Developed at Harvard Medical School*. New York: Owl Books, Henry Holt.

Khoury J. and Doghramji, K. (2015). Primary sleep disorders. *Psychiatric Clinics of North America*, **38** (4), 683–704.

Kripke, D. F., Langer, R. D., Elliott, J. A,. Klauber, M. R., and Rex, K. M. (2011). Mortality related to actigraphic long and short sleep. *Sleep Medicine*, **12**, 28–33.

Kripke, D. F., Langer, R. D., and Kline, L. E. (2012). Hypnotics' association with mortality or cancer: a matched cohort study. *BMJ, Open*, **2** (1), e000850.

Kyger, M. (2017). *The Mystery of Sleep: Why a Good Night's Rest Is Vital to a Better, Healthier Life*. Yale University press.

Morselli, L. L., Guyon A., and Spiegel, K. (2012). Sleep and metabolic function. *Pflügers Archiv - European Journal of Physiology*, **463** (1), 139–160.

National Code of Practice: For Managing Nurses' Fatigue and Shift Work in District Health Board Hospitals. (2019). *Safer Nursing, 24/7*, 1st edit, May 2019).

Nierenberg, A. A. (2016). Why we sleep. *Psychiatric Annals*, **4**(7), 381.

Paine, S.-J., Gander, P. H., Harris, R., and Reid, P. (2005). Prevalence and consequences of insomnia in New Zealand: disparities between Maori and non-Maori. *Australian and New Zealand Journal of Public Health*, **29** (1), 1–28.

Seber, G. A. F. (2013). *Counseling Issues: A Handbook for Counselors and Psychotherapists*. XLibris, and Wild Side publishing, New Zealand.

Seber, G. A. F. and Woodfield, D. G. (2020). *Alcohol: A Dangerous Love Affair*. Wild Side Publishing, New Zealand.

Stanley, N. (2018). *How to Sleep Well: The Science of Sleeping Smarter, Living Better and Being Productive*. Chichester: Wiley.

Walker, M. (2018). *Why We Sleep: Unlocking the Power of Sleep and Dreams*. New York: Scribner.

Wilsmore, B. R., Grunstein, R. R., Fransen, M., Woodward, M., Norton, R., and Ameratunga, S. (2013). Sleep habits, insomnia, and daytime sleepiness in a large and healthy community-based sample of New Zealanders. *Journal of Clinical Sleep Medicine*, **9** (6), 559–566.

OTHER BOOKS FROM GEORGE A.F. SEBER:

George Seber is also the author or co-author of seventeen books on statistics.

Alcohol: A dangerous love affair

All you need to know about alcohol.
An in-depth study of the effects of alcohol on users, the community, the nation of New Zealand, and globally.

ISBN: 978-0-473-50321-5

More books overleaf...

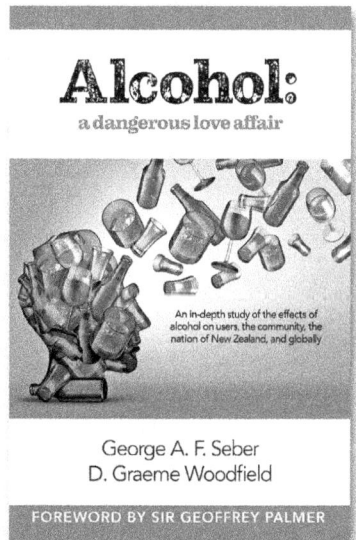

Alcohol:
a dangerous love affair

An in-depth study of the effects of alcohol on users, the community, the nation of New Zealand, and globally

George A. F. Seber
D. Graeme Woodfield

FOREWORD BY SIR GEOFFREY PALMER

OTHER BOOKS FROM GEORGE A.F. SEBER:

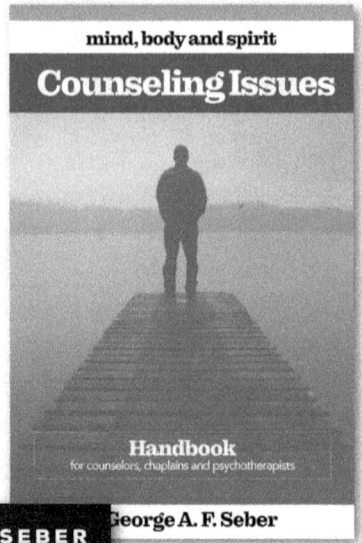

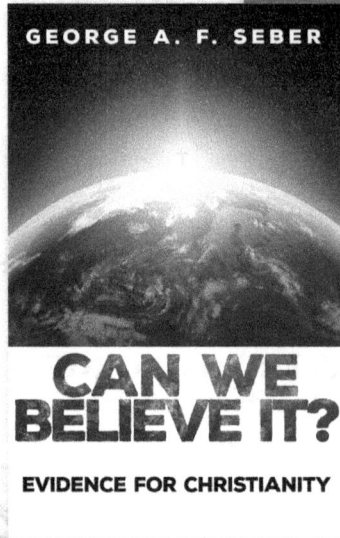

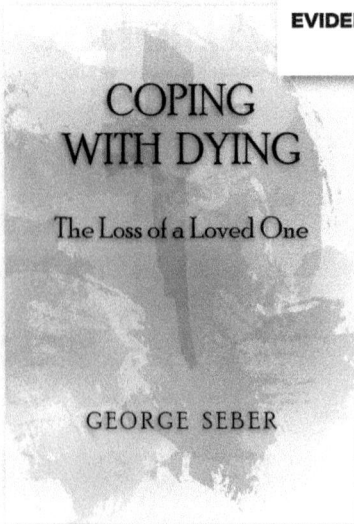

www.ingramcontent.com/pod-product-compliance
Lightning Source LLC
Chambersburg PA
CBHW072156020426
42334CB00018B/2027